KETO DIET TRACKER

KETO DIET
Tracker

AN 8-MONTH JOURNAL FOR EXERCISE, WEIGHT LOSS, MACROS, AND MORE

ROCKRIDGE
PRESS

For general information on our other products and services or to obtain technical support, please contact our Customer Care Department within the United States at (866) 744-2665, or outside the United States at (510) 253-0500.

Rockridge Press publishes its books in a variety of electronic and print formats. Some content that appears in print may not be available in electronic books, and vice versa.

Interior and Cover Designer: Irene Vandervoort
Art Producer: Alyssa Williams
Editor: Leah Zarra
Production Editor: Ashley Polikoff
Production Manager: Martin Worthington

All illustrations used under license from shutterstock.com

ISBN: 978-1-638-78934-5
R0

CONTENTS

INTRODUCTION

Welcome to your keto diet tracker! This journal is the
first step to mastering the keto diet and your weight-loss goals.
The keto diet, with its focus on the ratio of macronutrients—fats,
proteins, and carbohydrates—consumed daily, is a great tool for
weight loss.

Part 1 of this journal provides an overview of the ketogenic
diet with information and tips on keto basics, reaching and staying in ketosis, tracking macros, stocking your kitchen, and using
this journal to its maximum benefit. Remember that it takes time
to adjust to the keto diet, so don't be discouraged!

Part 2 is your keto diet tracker. It provides eight months of
daily, weekly, and monthly check-ins to log your macros and track
your weight loss.

While it can seem daunting at first, a food journal is a great tool
to use for all stages of your weight-loss journey, enabling you to
monitor your daily macros and see your progress over the months.
This journal also gives you the opportunity to reflect on and track
other aspects of your life beyond food, such as healthy habits, your
feelings, and exercise—all components of a healthy lifestyle!

Good luck and happy journaling!

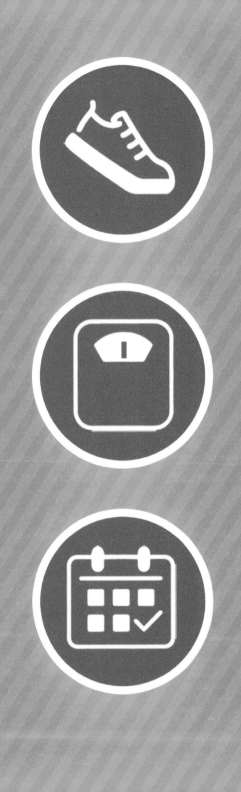

Part 1

GETTING
STARTED

In part 1, we'll cover all the essentials you need to know to begin the keto diet, from tracking macros, to staying in ketosis, to stocking your kitchen with keto-friendly foods. At the end, we'll explain how to use the journal in part 2 for daily, weekly, and monthly check-ins.

Unpacking the Keto Diet

What makes the ketogenic diet so unique is its emphasis on consuming a low-carb, high-fat diet and calculating macronutrients. Macronutrients, or macros, give you energy and are the basic building blocks of your diet. They are broken down into fats, proteins, and carbohydrates. On the keto diet, the goal is to have a daily caloric intake ratio of ~5% carbs, ~25% proteins, and ~70% fats. By doing this, your body will reach a metabolic state of "ketosis" where it burns fat instead of sugar/glucose (more on this later).

Maintaining this low-carb, high-fat diet is ideal for weight loss, and according to an increasing number of studies, it helps reduce risk factors for diabetes, heart disease, stroke, Alzheimer's, epilepsy, and more. The keto diet promotes fresh whole foods like meat, fish, veggies, and healthy fats and oils, and also greatly reduces processed, chemically treated foods, and refined grains and sugars.

Studies consistently show that a keto diet helps people lose more weight, improve energy levels throughout the day, and stay satiated longer.

When you eat a ketogenic diet, your body becomes efficient at burning fat for fuel. This is great for a multitude of reasons, not the least of which is that fat contains more than double the calories of most carbs, so you need to eat far less food by weight every day. Your body more readily burns the fat it has stored (the fat you're trying to get rid of), resulting in more weight loss. Using fat for fuel provides consistent energy levels, and it does not spike your blood glucose, so you don't experience the highs and lows you would when eating large amounts of carbs. Consistent energy levels throughout your day means you can get more done and feel less tired doing so.

How to Reach and Stay in Ketosis

In the typical high-carb diet, your body is in a metabolic state of glycolysis, which simply means that most of the energy your body uses comes from blood glucose. In contrast, a low-carb, high-fat diet like keto puts your body into a metabolic state called *ketosis*. With this diet, your body breaks down fat into ketone bodies (ketones) for fuel as its primary source of energy. In ketosis, your body readily burns fat for energy, and fat reserves are constantly released and consumed. It's a normal state and whenever you're low on carbs for a few days, your body will do this naturally.

Getting into and staying in ketosis is the goal with keto, and the best way to get there is by restricting your carbohydrates and upping your fat intake. To reach ketosis and start burning fat, your body must first burn through its stored glucose/sugar. That process can take as little as two to four days or sometimes longer. Some great signs that you're in ketosis are weight loss or a decreased appetite. Another weird but equally great sign of ketosis is having a funky, fruity taste in your mouth—welcome to ketosis!

When first entering ketosis, some people may experience short-term symptoms such as nausea or feeling run-down, even sick. This is often called the "keto flu." These symptoms tend to be mild and are usually caused by the loss of water weight and electrolytes in the first few days. Many folks give up at this point, but if you can stick it out, you'll find that the keto flu doesn't last long. Push past the symptoms by replacing those lost electrolytes with supplements. Drink more water, sugar-free electrolyte sports drinks, or warm bone broth.

Knowing Your Macros

Tracking your macros—fats, proteins, and carbohydrates—is the key to success on the keto diet. For the ideal ratio, 65 to 75 percent of the calories you consume should come from fat, about 20 to 25 percent from protein, and the remaining 5 percent or so from carbohydrates. Monitoring and adhering to these ratios are what make the keto diet seem so strict, but you'll see that you can still enjoy many of your favorite foods.

FATS

Consuming foods with 75 percent fat or higher is the easiest way to reach your keto goal of ketosis and weight loss. While some fats are healthier than others, all fats are beneficial in some way, whether it's unsaturated fats found in foods like avocados, nuts, and olive oils, or saturated fats found in foods like butter, red meat, and eggs. There are some unhealthy fat sources to stay away from, including processed trans fats and vegetable oils (oils extracted from seeds), such as corn, canola, grapeseed, peanut, soybean, and sunflower oils, margarine, and vegetable shortening.

PROTEINS

For keto, the goal is to keep protein around 20 to 25 percent of your total calories. The body converts excess protein into glucose, a process called *gluconeogenesis*, which can potentially kick you out of ketosis. But protein also keeps you full, supports strong bones, and builds a strong immune system. Unlike fats and carbs, protein isn't stored in the body, so it's important to get enough protein every day. A great way to stay in balance with fat and protein is to eat fattier cuts of meat, such as beef ribeye, New York strip steak, chicken thighs, pork ribs, and hamburger meat. Lean meats like skinless chicken, turkey, beef, and pork are also good, but you'll need to compensate with fat elsewhere to meet your goal.

CARBOHYDRATES

Restricting carb intake is a must on the keto diet. Generally, you should be eating around 20 to 50 grams of carbs per day (5 to 10 percent of calories). Some people may be able to eat additional carbs and stay in ketosis, whereas others might need to cut back.

This journal will log net carbs rather than total carbs. "Total carbs" refers to all the carbs that a serving of food contains, and "net carbs" are the actual carbs absorbed by the body that have an impact on your blood sugar. To calculate the net carbs of a whole food, such as a piece of fruit, subtract the fiber from the total amount of carbs—fiber doesn't get used in the body because it doesn't break down, so it can be deducted.

UNDERSTANDING YOUR MACRO RATIOS

The energy from the three macronutrients can be quantified by this equation: **carbs + protein + fat = total calories**. Depending on your individual goals, macros can be tracked as percentages of the food you eat every day. Each person's target macros may be different, so you'll want to figure out your individual macro needs.

To do this, you can go online and search "macro calculators." There are many available free of charge. You'll be able to enter information such as your height, weight, gender, exercise levels, and weight-loss goals, and they'll calculate optimal macros for whatever goals you have. It's important to determine your desired daily calorie intake as this will inform macronutrient calculations. Then, you'll want 70 to 75 percent of your daily calories to come from fat, 20 to 25 percent to come from protein, and 5 to 10 percent to come from carbs.

When tracking your macros for each meal, consult the food's nutritional labels or the USDA Nutrient Analysis Library to determine the grams for each macro. As each type of macronutrient provides a certain amount of energy (calories) per gram consumed (fat = 9 calories per gram, protein = 4 calories per gram, and carbs = 4 calories per gram), there are quick formulas to convert from grams to percentage of daily calories:

- Percentage Fat = ((Total grams × 9) / Total Daily Calories) × 100

- Percentage Protein = ((Total grams × 4) / Total Daily Calories) × 100

- Percentage Carbohydrates = ((Total grams × 4) / Total Daily Calories) × 100

How to Eat on the Keto Diet

Now that you understand how the body works with regard to keto, let's explore the food! Keto focuses on eating high-quality whole foods that are minimally processed or preserved to achieve ketosis. While the idea of drastically reducing your carb intake can seem daunting, there are so many flavorful and delicious foods to try. Remember that although it may seem tempting to load up on protein and ignore portion sizes, doing so can lead to weight-loss struggles or even gains. Keep a balanced plate with a healthy mix of proteins and low-carb vegetables and fruits.

On page 7 you'll find a short chart of foods to enjoy and avoid on the keto diet. Note that unlike other diets, food categories such as vegetables and fruits are included under both, so be sure to double-check the specific food you're eating.

FOODS TO ENJOY AND AVOID
ON THE KETO DIET

FOODS TO ENJOY	FOODS TO AVOID
Meat (bacon, chicken, deli meats, ham, hot dogs, pepperoni, pork, pork belly, pork rinds, prosciutto, salami, sausage, turkey, veal)	Proteins (breaded meats, deli meats and hot dogs with added sugars, glazed ham, imitation crab meat)
Fish (clams, cod, flounder, herring, lobster, oysters, salmon, sardines, shrimp, sole, tilapia, tuna)	Dairy (condensed milk, custards, milk, puddings, sweet milks, yogurt)
Eggs	Sugary Foods
Dairy (bread cheese, butter, cream cheese, ghee, hard cheeses, heavy cream, mascarpone, soft cheeses, sour cream, string cheese)	Grains or Starches (barley, bread, brown rice, cookies, corn tortillas, crackers, flour tortillas, oatmeal, pasta, quinoa, white rice)
Fruit (avocados, blackberries, blueberries, lemons, limes, olives, raspberries, strawberries, tomatoes, unsweetened coconut)	Fruit (apples, bananas, canned fruits, dried fruits, fruit juices, mangos, oranges, peaches, pears, pineapples)
Nuts & Seeds (chia seeds, flaxseed, hemp seeds, sesame seeds)	Beans or Legumes
	Vegetables (carrots, corn, parsnips, peas, potatoes, sweet pickles, sweet potatoes, yams)
Healthy Oils (olive oil, coconut oil, avocado oil)	Low-Fat or Diet Products
Low-Carb Veggies (asparagus, cabbage, celery, chives, cucumbers, eggplant, green chiles, kale, leafy greens, mushrooms, pickles, radishes, spinach, zucchini)	Alcohol
	Sugar-Free Diet Foods
Salt and Pepper	
Herbs and Spices	

HOW TO BEAT THE "KETO FLU"

The "keto flu" is avoidable, and its duration can be reduced simply by adding more sodium to your diet. Here are some of the easiest ways to do that:

- Add more salt to your meals.

- Drink soup broths like beef and chicken.

- Eat saltier foods like pickled vegetables and bacon.

To replace other electrolytes, try to eat more of the foods listed below:

ELECTROLYTE	FOODS CONTAINING ELECTROLYTE
POTASSIUM	Avocados, dark leafy greens such as spinach and kale, mushrooms, nuts, plain yogurt, salmon
MAGNESIUM	Artichokes, dark chocolate, fish, nuts, spinach
CALCIUM	Almonds, broccoli, cheeses, leafy greens, seafood
PHOSPHORUS	Cheeses, dark chocolate, meats, nuts, seeds
CHLORIDE	Most vegetables, olives, salt, seaweed

Remember that if you don't feel better right away, the flu will pass within a couple of days, and you'll emerge a fat-burning machine!

Additional Tips for Success

While the keto diet is great for weight loss, there are a few other factors that can aid in your weight-loss journey. You'll see that the daily entries in this journal provide space to track your water intake, sleep, and exercise.

Water: Water is a great weight-loss tool and necessary on the keto diet because dehydration is a common side effect of ketosis. Your body is used to eating carbs and storing that energy as glycogen (the stored form of glucose). When you restrict carbs and burn through all your stored glucose, you lose a great deal of water weight and electrolytes in the process, so aim to drink at least eight 8-ounce glasses of water per day.

Sleep: Poor sleep can result in increased appetite and weight gain, which in turn makes it harder to sleep going forward. Aim for 6 to 8 hours of sleep per night.

Exercise: Exercise is a great companion to the keto diet as it will further boost weight-loss success. For beginners, start taking short walks or slow jogs for 15 minutes every other day. If you already go to the gym or lift weights, add an extra exercise. It doesn't matter what level you're at; just try to do a little more than you're doing now.

Limit Alcohol: While you can still consume alcohol on the keto diet, it's best practice to limit the amount and type. Substitute sugary cocktails like piña coladas and margaritas for an occasional low-carb beer or glass of white wine, or liquors such as vodka, whiskey, tequila, or rum.

How to Use This Journal

Weight-loss journals are a valuable tool for the keto diet, as there's so much to track. As keto requires tracking macros for each meal plus daily and weekly totals, having a space to record and monitor is essential. Using a journal is also beneficial because it increases your awareness of your lifestyle choices and habits by giving you room to write down what you're eating, monitor your macros intake, note how you feel after consuming different foods, and make informed, conscious decisions for the day and week ahead.

This journal will help you along your weight-loss journey through daily, weekly, and monthly reporting and reflection. While the daily and weekly entries are focused on eating, macros, and moods, the monthly check-ins enable you to track your weight-loss progress. In addition, all the dates for the entries are blank for greater flexibility so you can start journaling on your time frame.

DAILY AND WEEKLY ENTRIES

For each week, there will be a four-page spread of seven daily entries to log meals and associated macros, water intake, exercise, mood, and sleep. Space is included for you to write your breakfast, lunch, dinner, and snacks consumed every day, and a sample entry has been included.

When completing the entries, here are some helpful tips:

- Note at what time you consume food. (It's best to try to eat every 3 to 4 hours.)

- Include the food quantity, even if it's just a quick estimate such as "handful of nuts."

- Complete your log after every meal, glass of water, or activity so you don't miss anything throughout the course of the day.

- Jot down notes throughout the day on how you're feeling, particularly if you notice any mood changes or drops in energy.

At the end of each week, you'll find reflection questions to assess the week and create action steps. Use these questions to celebrate what you did well each week, such as hitting your macro goals, while also determining what you can improve the next week, like drinking more water if you felt dehydrated or choosing to eat more whole foods. Remember this is your journal, so use it however best aids your diet!

SAMPLE DAILY ENTRY

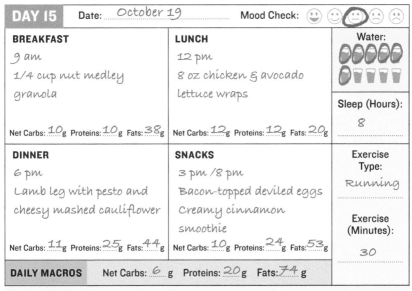

DAY 15 Date: *October 19* Mood Check: 🙂 🙂 😐 🙁 ☹

BREAKFAST	LUNCH	Water:
9 am	*12 pm*	🍶🍶🍶🍶🍶
1/4 cup nut medley granola	*8 oz chicken & avocado lettuce wraps*	🍶🥛🥛🥛🥛
		Sleep (Hours):
Net Carbs: *10* g Proteins: *10* g Fats: *38* g	Net Carbs: *12* g Proteins: *12* g Fats: *20* g	*8*
DINNER	**SNACKS**	**Exercise Type:**
6 pm	*3 pm / 8 pm*	*Running*
Lamb leg with pesto and cheesy mashed cauliflower	*Bacon-topped deviled eggs Creamy cinnamon smoothie*	**Exercise (Minutes):**
Net Carbs: *11* g Proteins: *25* g Fats: *44* g	Net Carbs: *10* g Proteins: *24* g Fats: *53* g	*30*
DAILY MACROS	Net Carbs: *6* g Proteins: *20* g Fats: *74* g	

Notes: *It was cold this morning, but I went for a run and felt fierce (and a little smug!) all day. I'm also feeling more control over cravings. I got this!*

4-WEEK CHECK-IN

At the start of the journal, you'll find a chart to log your initial weight and body measurements for your upper arms, chest, waist, hips, thighs, and calves. Here are some tips for where (and how) to measure:

- Upper arms—Bend your elbow. Flex your arm and measure your bicep.

- Chest—Measure the widest part around your bust or chest.

- Waist—Measure the narrowest part of your torso.

- Hips—Measure the widest part of your glutes (your butt muscle).

- Thighs—Measure the midpoint between the lower glutes and the back of your knee.

- Calves—Measure halfway between your knee and your ankle.

Every four weeks there will be a check-in with the same chart to assess your progress on your weight-loss goals. This chart will also include an additional column to note your progress (decreases, no change, or increases). Beneath each chart is a series of questions to reflect on your progress and set new goals. Remember, don't be distressed if you don't immediately lose weight—everyone moves at their own pace!

While you can check your own progress in between each four-week check-in, your weight fluctuates day to day, so measuring over a longer time span will give you more realistic and impactful results. When weighing and measuring yourself, remember to always do so at the same time of day (morning is usually best) and the same way for the most consistent and precise numbers.

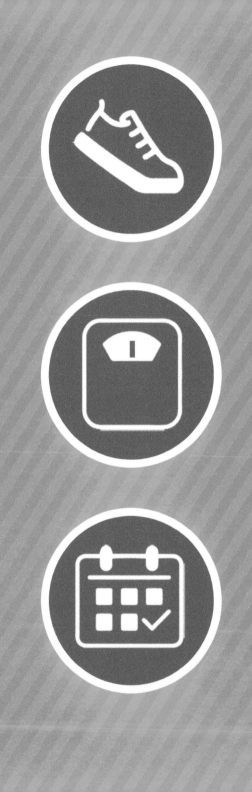

Part 2

TRACKING YOUR KETO DIET

Welcome to part 2—your keto weight-loss journal! For the next eight months, these pages will allow you to record your daily, weekly, and monthly numbers and progress. Remember that weight loss is different for every person, so use this journal to celebrate your achievements at your pace.

BASELINE CHECK-IN

MEASUREMENT	CURRENT
WEIGHT (LBS)	
UPPER ARMS (IN)	
CHEST (IN)	
WAIST (IN)	
HIPS (IN)	
THIGHS (IN)	
CALVES (IN)	

WEEKLY INTENTIONS

What are you excited for this week?

TARGET MACROS
Carbs: .... %
Proteins: .... %
Fats: .... %

....

....

....

What is something you'd like to work on this week? ....

....

....

....

DAY 1 Date: .... Mood Check: 😃 🙂 😐 🙁 😣

BREAKFAST	LUNCH	Water:
		🥤🥤🥤🥤🥤
		🥤🥤🥤🥤🥤
		Sleep (Hours):
Net Carbs: ...... g Proteins: ...... g Fats: ...... g	Net Carbs: ...... g Proteins: ...... g Fats: ...... g	....
DINNER	**SNACKS**	Exercise Type:
		....
		Exercise (Minutes):
Net Carbs: ...... g Proteins: ...... g Fats: ...... g	Net Carbs: ...... g Proteins: ...... g Fats: ...... g	....
DAILY MACROS Net Carbs: ...... g Proteins: ...... g Fats: ...... g		

Notes:

DAY 2

Date: .... Mood Check: 😀 🙂 😐 🙁 😣

BREAKFAST	LUNCH	Water:
		🥛🥛🥛🥛🥛 🥛🥛🥛🥛🥛
		Sleep (Hours):
Net Carbs: ...... g Proteins: ...... g Fats: ...... g	Net Carbs: ...... g Proteins: ...... g Fats: ...... g	....
DINNER	**SNACKS**	Exercise Type:
		....
		Exercise (Minutes):
Net Carbs: ...... g Proteins: ...... g Fats: ...... g	Net Carbs: ...... g Proteins: ...... g Fats: ...... g	....
DAILY MACROS Net Carbs: ...... g Proteins: ...... g Fats: ...... g		

Notes:

DAY 3

Date: .... Mood Check: 😀 🙂 😐 🙁 😣

BREAKFAST	LUNCH	Water:
		🥛🥛🥛🥛🥛 🥛🥛🥛🥛🥛
		Sleep (Hours):
Net Carbs: ...... g Proteins: ...... g Fats: ...... g	Net Carbs: ...... g Proteins: ...... g Fats: ...... g	....
DINNER	**SNACKS**	Exercise Type:
		....
		Exercise (Minutes):
Net Carbs: ...... g Proteins: ...... g Fats: ...... g	Net Carbs: ...... g Proteins: ...... g Fats: ...... g	....
DAILY MACROS Net Carbs: ...... g Proteins: ...... g Fats: ...... g		

Notes:

DAY 4   Date: ....   Mood Check: 😀 😊 😐 😕 😖

BREAKFAST	LUNCH	Water:
		🥤🥤🥤🥤🥤 🥤🥤🥤🥤🥤
		Sleep (Hours):
Net Carbs: ...... g Proteins: ...... g Fats: ...... g	Net Carbs: ...... g Proteins: ...... g Fats: ...... g	....
DINNER	SNACKS	Exercise Type:
		....
		Exercise (Minutes):
Net Carbs: ...... g Proteins: ...... g Fats: ...... g	Net Carbs: ...... g Proteins: ...... g Fats: ...... g	....

DAILY MACROS   Net Carbs: .... g   Proteins: .... g   Fats: .... g

Notes:

DAY 5   Date: ....   Mood Check: 😀 😊 😐 😕 😖

BREAKFAST	LUNCH	Water:
		🥤🥤🥤🥤🥤 🥤🥤🥤🥤🥤
		Sleep (Hours):
Net Carbs: ...... g Proteins: ...... g Fats: ...... g	Net Carbs: ...... g Proteins: ...... g Fats: ...... g	....
DINNER	SNACKS	Exercise Type:
		....
		Exercise (Minutes):
Net Carbs: ...... g Proteins: ...... g Fats: ...... g	Net Carbs: ...... g Proteins: ...... g Fats: ...... g	....

DAILY MACROS   Net Carbs: .... g   Proteins: .... g   Fats: .... g

Notes:

DAY 6   Date: ....   Mood Check: 😀 😊 😐 🙁 ☹️

BREAKFAST	LUNCH	Water:
		🥛🥛🥛🥛 🥛🥛🥛🥛
		Sleep (Hours):
Net Carbs: ...... g Proteins: ...... g Fats: ...... g	Net Carbs: ...... g Proteins: ...... g Fats: ...... g	....
DINNER	**SNACKS**	Exercise Type:
		....
		Exercise (Minutes):
Net Carbs: ...... g Proteins: ...... g Fats: ...... g	Net Carbs: ...... g Proteins: ...... g Fats: ...... g	....
DAILY MACROS Net Carbs: ...... g Proteins: ...... g Fats: ...... g		

Notes:

DAY 7   Date: ....   Mood Check: 😀 😊 😐 🙁 ☹️

BREAKFAST	LUNCH	Water:
		🥛🥛🥛🥛 🥛🥛🥛🥛
		Sleep (Hours):
Net Carbs: ...... g Proteins: ...... g Fats: ...... g	Net Carbs: ...... g Proteins: ...... g Fats: ...... g	....
DINNER	**SNACKS**	Exercise Type:
		....
		Exercise (Minutes):
Net Carbs: ...... g Proteins: ...... g Fats: ...... g	Net Carbs: ...... g Proteins: ...... g Fats: ...... g	....
DAILY MACROS Net Carbs: ...... g Proteins: ...... g Fats: ...... g		

Notes:

WEEKLY INTENTIONS

What are you excited for this week?

....

....

....

....

What is something you'd like to work on this week? ....

....

....

....

Carbs: .... %
Proteins: .... %
Fats: .... %

DAY 8	Date:	Mood Check: ☺ ☺ ☺ ☹ ☹

BREAKFAST	LUNCH	Water:
		🥛🥛🥛🥛🥛 🥛🥛🥛🥛🥛
		Sleep (Hours):
Net Carbs: ...... g Proteins: ...... g Fats: ...... g	Net Carbs: ...... g Proteins: ...... g Fats: ...... g	....
DINNER	SNACKS	Exercise Type: ....
		Exercise (Minutes):
Net Carbs: ...... g Proteins: ...... g Fats: ...... g	Net Carbs: ...... g Proteins: ...... g Fats: ...... g	....
DAILY MACROS	Net Carbs: ...... g Proteins: ...... g Fats: ...... g	

Notes:

DAY 9

Date: .... Mood Check: 😀 🙂 😐 🙁 😧

BREAKFAST	LUNCH	Water:
		🥛🥛🥛🥛🥛 🥛🥛🥛🥛🥛
		Sleep (Hours):
Net Carbs: ...... g Proteins: ...... g Fats: ...... g	Net Carbs: ...... g Proteins: ...... g Fats: ...... g	....
DINNER	**SNACKS**	Exercise Type: .... Exercise (Minutes):
Net Carbs: ...... g Proteins: ...... g Fats: ...... g	Net Carbs: ...... g Proteins: ...... g Fats: ...... g	....

DAILY MACROS   Net Carbs: ...... g   Proteins: ...... g   Fats: ...... g

Notes:

DAY 10

Date: .... Mood Check: 😀 🙂 😐 🙁 😧

BREAKFAST	LUNCH	Water:
		🥛🥛🥛🥛🥛 🥛🥛🥛🥛🥛
		Sleep (Hours):
Net Carbs: ...... g Proteins: ...... g Fats: ...... g	Net Carbs: ...... g Proteins: ...... g Fats: ...... g	....
DINNER	**SNACKS**	Exercise Type: .... Exercise (Minutes):
Net Carbs: ...... g Proteins: ...... g Fats: ...... g	Net Carbs: ...... g Proteins: ...... g Fats: ...... g	....

DAILY MACROS   Net Carbs: ...... g   Proteins: ...... g   Fats: ...... g

Notes:

DAY 11 Date: .... Mood Check: 😀 😊 😐 😟 😧

BREAKFAST	LUNCH	Water:
		🥤🥤🥤🥤🥤 🥤🥤🥤🥤🥤
		Sleep (Hours):
Net Carbs: ...... g Proteins: ...... g Fats: ...... g	Net Carbs: ...... g Proteins: ...... g Fats: ...... g	....
DINNER	SNACKS	Exercise Type:
		....
		Exercise (Minutes):
Net Carbs: ...... g Proteins: ...... g Fats: ...... g	Net Carbs: ...... g Proteins: ...... g Fats: ...... g	....

DAILY MACROS   Net Carbs: .... g   Proteins: .... g   Fats: .... g

Notes:

DAY 12 Date: .... Mood Check: 😀 😊 😐 😟 😧

BREAKFAST	LUNCH	Water:
		🥤🥤🥤🥤🥤 🥤🥤🥤🥤🥤
		Sleep (Hours):
Net Carbs: ...... g Proteins: ...... g Fats: ...... g	Net Carbs: ...... g Proteins: ...... g Fats: ...... g	....
DINNER	SNACKS	Exercise Type:
		....
		Exercise (Minutes):
Net Carbs: ...... g Proteins: ...... g Fats: ...... g	Net Carbs: ...... g Proteins: ...... g Fats: ...... g	....

DAILY MACROS   Net Carbs: .... g   Proteins: .... g   Fats: .... g

Notes:

DAY 13　Date: ....　Mood Check: 😊 🙂 😐 🙁 😣

BREAKFAST	LUNCH	Water:
		🥤🥤🥤🥤🥤 🥤🥤🥤🥤🥤
		Sleep (Hours):
Net Carbs: ...... g Proteins: ...... g Fats: ...... g	Net Carbs: ...... g Proteins: ...... g Fats: ...... g	....
DINNER	SNACKS	Exercise Type: ....
		Exercise (Minutes):
Net Carbs: ...... g Proteins: ...... g Fats: ...... g	Net Carbs: ...... g Proteins: ...... g Fats: ...... g	....
DAILY MACROS　Net Carbs: ...... g　Proteins: ...... g　Fats: ...... g		

Notes:

DAY 14　Date: ....　Mood Check: 😊 🙂 😐 🙁 😣

BREAKFAST	LUNCH	Water:
		🥤🥤🥤🥤🥤 🥤🥤🥤🥤🥤
		Sleep (Hours):
Net Carbs: ...... g Proteins: ...... g Fats: ...... g	Net Carbs: ...... g Proteins: ...... g Fats: ...... g	....
DINNER	SNACKS	Exercise Type: ....
		Exercise (Minutes):
Net Carbs: ...... g Proteins: ...... g Fats: ...... g	Net Carbs: ...... g Proteins: ...... g Fats: ...... g	....
DAILY MACROS　Net Carbs: ...... g　Proteins: ...... g　Fats: ...... g		

Notes:

WEEKLY INTENTIONS

What are you excited for this week?

....

....

....

....

What is something you'd like to work on this week? ....

....

....

....

TARGET MACROS

Carbs: .... %
Proteins: .... %
Fats: .... %

DAY 15   Date: ....   Mood Check: 😀 😊 😐 😕 😣

BREAKFAST	LUNCH	Water:
		🥤🥤🥤🥤🥤 🥤🥤🥤🥤🥤
		Sleep (Hours):
Net Carbs: ...... g Proteins: ...... g Fats: ...... g	Net Carbs: ...... g Proteins: ...... g Fats: ...... g	....
DINNER	**SNACKS**	Exercise Type:
		....
		Exercise (Minutes):
Net Carbs: ...... g Proteins: ...... g Fats: ...... g	Net Carbs: ...... g Proteins: ...... g Fats: ...... g	....

DAILY MACROS   Net Carbs: ...... g   Proteins: ...... g   Fats: ...... g

Notes:

DAY 16

Date: .... Mood Check: 😄 ☺ 😐 🙁 ☹

BREAKFAST	LUNCH	Water:
		🥛🥛🥛🥛🥛 🥛🥛🥛🥛🥛
		Sleep (Hours):
Net Carbs: ...... g Proteins: ...... g Fats: ...... g	Net Carbs: ...... g Proteins: ...... g Fats: ...... g	....
DINNER	SNACKS	Exercise Type:
		....
		Exercise (Minutes):
Net Carbs: ...... g Proteins: ...... g Fats: ...... g	Net Carbs: ...... g Proteins: ...... g Fats: ...... g	....

DAILY MACROS   Net Carbs: ...... g   Proteins: ...... g   Fats: ...... g

Notes:

DAY 17

Date: .... Mood Check: 😄 ☺ 😐 🙁 ☹

BREAKFAST	LUNCH	Water:
		🥛🥛🥛🥛🥛 🥛🥛🥛🥛🥛
		Sleep (Hours):
Net Carbs: ...... g Proteins: ...... g Fats: ...... g	Net Carbs: ...... g Proteins: ...... g Fats: ...... g	....
DINNER	SNACKS	Exercise Type:
		....
		Exercise (Minutes):
Net Carbs: ...... g Proteins: ...... g Fats: ...... g	Net Carbs: ...... g Proteins: ...... g Fats: ...... g	....

DAILY MACROS   Net Carbs: ...... g   Proteins: ...... g   Fats: ...... g

Notes:

DAY 18   Date: ....   Mood Check: 😀 🙂 😐 🙁 😧

BREAKFAST

LUNCH

Water:

Sleep (Hours):

Net Carbs: ...... g Proteins: ...... g Fats: ...... g | Net Carbs: ...... g Proteins: ...... g Fats: ...... g

....

DINNER

SNACKS

Exercise Type:

....

Exercise (Minutes):

Net Carbs: ...... g Proteins: ...... g Fats: ...... g | Net Carbs: ...... g Proteins: ...... g Fats: ...... g

....

DAILY MACROS   Net Carbs: ...... g   Proteins: ...... g   Fats: ...... g

Notes:

DAY 19   Date: ....   Mood Check: 😀 🙂 😐 🙁 😧

BREAKFAST

LUNCH

Water:

Sleep (Hours):

Net Carbs: ...... g Proteins: ...... g Fats: ...... g | Net Carbs: ...... g Proteins: ...... g Fats: ...... g

....

DINNER

SNACKS

Exercise Type:

....

Exercise (Minutes):

Net Carbs: ...... g Proteins: ...... g Fats: ...... g | Net Carbs: ...... g Proteins: ...... g Fats: ...... g

....

DAILY MACROS   Net Carbs: ...... g   Proteins: ...... g   Fats: ...... g

Notes:

DAY 20 Date:.. Mood Check: 😊 🙂 😐 😕 ☹️

BREAKFAST	LUNCH	Water:
		🥛🥛🥛🥛🥛 🥛🥛🥛🥛🥛
		Sleep (Hours):
Net Carbs: ...... g Proteins: ...... g Fats: ...... g	Net Carbs: ...... g Proteins: ...... g Fats: ...... g	....
DINNER	SNACKS	Exercise Type:
		....
		Exercise (Minutes):
Net Carbs: ...... g Proteins: ...... g Fats: ...... g	Net Carbs: ...... g Proteins: ...... g Fats: ...... g	....
DAILY MACROS	Net Carbs: ...... g Proteins: ...... g Fats: ...... g	

Notes:

DAY 21 Date:.. Mood Check: 😊 🙂 😐 😕 ☹️

BREAKFAST	LUNCH	Water:
		🥛🥛🥛🥛🥛 🥛🥛🥛🥛🥛
		Sleep (Hours):
Net Carbs: ...... g Proteins: ...... g Fats: ...... g	Net Carbs: ...... g Proteins: ...... g Fats: ...... g	....
DINNER	SNACKS	Exercise Type:
		....
		Exercise (Minutes):
Net Carbs: ...... g Proteins: ...... g Fats: ...... g	Net Carbs: ...... g Proteins: ...... g Fats: ...... g	....
DAILY MACROS	Net Carbs: ...... g Proteins: ...... g Fats: ...... g	

Notes:

WEEKLY INTENTIONS

What are you excited for this week?

....

....

....

What is something you'd like to work on this week? ....

....

....

....

Carbs: .... %
Proteins: .... %
Fats: .... %

DAY 22	Date:	Mood Check: 😀 🙂 😐 🙁 😣
BREAKFAST	**LUNCH**	Water:
		Sleep (Hours):
Net Carbs: ...... g Proteins: ...... g Fats: ...... g	Net Carbs: ...... g Proteins: ...... g Fats: ...... g	....
DINNER	**SNACKS**	Exercise Type:
		....
		Exercise (Minutes):
Net Carbs: ...... g Proteins: ...... g Fats: ...... g	Net Carbs: ...... g Proteins: ...... g Fats: ...... g	....
DAILY MACROS	Net Carbs: ...... g Proteins: ...... g Fats: ...... g	

Notes:

DAY 23　Date: ....　Mood Check: 😀 😊 😐 😟 😣

BREAKFAST	LUNCH	Water:
		🥛🥛🥛🥛🥛 🥛🥛🥛🥛🥛
		Sleep (Hours):
Net Carbs: ...... g Proteins: ...... g Fats: ...... g	Net Carbs: ...... g Proteins: ...... g Fats: ...... g	....
DINNER	**SNACKS**	Exercise Type: .... Exercise (Minutes):
Net Carbs: ...... g Proteins: ...... g Fats: ...... g	Net Carbs: ...... g Proteins: ...... g Fats: ...... g	....
DAILY MACROS　Net Carbs: ...... g　Proteins: ...... g　Fats: ...... g		

Notes:

DAY 24　Date: ....　Mood Check: 😀 😊 😐 😟 😣

BREAKFAST	LUNCH	Water:
		🥛🥛🥛🥛🥛 🥛🥛🥛🥛🥛
		Sleep (Hours):
Net Carbs: ...... g Proteins: ...... g Fats: ...... g	Net Carbs: ...... g Proteins: ...... g Fats: ...... g	....
DINNER	**SNACKS**	Exercise Type: .... Exercise (Minutes):
Net Carbs: ...... g Proteins: ...... g Fats: ...... g	Net Carbs: ...... g Proteins: ...... g Fats: ...... g	....
DAILY MACROS　Net Carbs: ...... g　Proteins: ...... g　Fats: ...... g		

Notes:

DAY 25

Date: .... Mood Check: 😀 😊 😐 😕 😣

BREAKFAST

LUNCH

Water:

🥛🥛🥛🥛🥛
🥛🥛🥛🥛🥛

Sleep (Hours):

Net Carbs: ...... g Proteins: ...... g Fats: ...... g | Net Carbs: ...... g Proteins: ...... g Fats: ...... g | ....

DINNER

SNACKS

Exercise
Type:

....

Exercise
(Minutes):

Net Carbs: ...... g Proteins: ...... g Fats: ...... g | Net Carbs: ...... g Proteins: ...... g Fats: ...... g | ....

DAILY MACROS   Net Carbs: ...... g   Proteins: ...... g   Fats: ...... g

Notes:

DAY 26

Date: .... Mood Check: 😀 😊 😐 😕 😣

BREAKFAST

LUNCH

Water:

🥛🥛🥛🥛🥛
🥛🥛🥛🥛🥛

Sleep (Hours):

Net Carbs: ...... g Proteins: ...... g Fats: ...... g | Net Carbs: ...... g Proteins: ...... g Fats: ...... g | ....

DINNER

SNACKS

Exercise
Type:

....

Exercise
(Minutes):

Net Carbs: ...... g Proteins: ...... g Fats: ...... g | Net Carbs: ...... g Proteins: ...... g Fats: ...... g | ....

DAILY MACROS   Net Carbs: ...... g   Proteins: ...... g   Fats: ...... g

Notes:

DAY 27   Date: ....   Mood Check: 😀 🙂 😐 😕 ☹️

BREAKFAST	LUNCH	Water: 🥤🥤🥤🥤🥤 🥤🥤🥤🥤🥤
		Sleep (Hours):
Net Carbs: ...... g Proteins: ...... g Fats: ...... g	Net Carbs: ...... g Proteins: ...... g Fats: ...... g	....
DINNER	**SNACKS**	Exercise Type: .... Exercise (Minutes):
Net Carbs: ...... g Proteins: ...... g Fats: ...... g	Net Carbs: ...... g Proteins: ...... g Fats: ...... g	....

DAILY MACROS   Net Carbs: .... g   Proteins: .... g   Fats: .... g

Notes:

DAY 28   Date: ....   Mood Check: 😀 🙂 😐 😕 ☹️

BREAKFAST	LUNCH	Water: 🥤🥤🥤🥤🥤 🥤🥤🥤🥤🥤
		Sleep (Hours):
Net Carbs: ...... g Proteins: ...... g Fats: ...... g	Net Carbs: ...... g Proteins: ...... g Fats: ...... g	....
DINNER	**SNACKS**	Exercise Type: .... Exercise (Minutes):
Net Carbs: ...... g Proteins: ...... g Fats: ...... g	Net Carbs: ...... g Proteins: ...... g Fats: ...... g	....

DAILY MACROS   Net Carbs: .... g   Proteins: .... g   Fats: .... g

Notes:

MEASUREMENT	CURRENT	MONTH CHANGE
WEIGHT (LBS)		
UPPER ARMS (IN)		
CHEST (IN)		
WAIST (IN)		
HIPS (IN)		
THIGHS (IN)		
CALVES (IN)		

CHECKING IN

Congratulations on making it this far! What are you most proud of from the past 4 weeks?

....

....

....

....

....

What was your biggest challenge over the past 4 weeks?

....

....

....

....

....

....

What are some goals you would like to work toward over the
next 4 weeks?

....

....

....

....

....

Reflect on your mood over the past month—did you notice
differences related to your eating habits?

....

....

....

....

....

WEEKLY INTENTIONS

What are you excited for this week?

....

....

....

What is something you'd like to work on this week? ....

....

....

....

TARGET MACROS

Carbs: .... %
Proteins: .... %
Fats: .... %

DAY 29	Date:	Mood Check: 😀 😊 😐 🙁 😞

BREAKFAST

LUNCH

Water:

Sleep (Hours):

Net Carbs: ...... g Proteins: ...... g Fats: ...... g

Net Carbs: ...... g Proteins: ...... g Fats: ...... g

DINNER

SNACKS

Exercise Type:

....

Exercise (Minutes):

Net Carbs: ...... g Proteins: ...... g Fats: ...... g

Net Carbs: ...... g Proteins: ...... g Fats: ...... g

DAILY MACROS   Net Carbs: ...... g   Proteins: ...... g   Fats: ...... g

Notes:

DAY 30	Date:	Mood Check: ☺ ☺ 😐 ☹ 😖

BREAKFAST	LUNCH	Water:
		🥤🥤🥤🥤🥤 🥤🥤🥤🥤🥤
		Sleep (Hours):
Net Carbs: ..... g Proteins: ..... g Fats: ..... g	Net Carbs: ..... g Proteins: ..... g Fats: ..... g	....

DINNER	SNACKS	Exercise Type:
		....
		Exercise (Minutes):
Net Carbs: ..... g Proteins: ..... g Fats: ..... g	Net Carbs: ..... g Proteins: ..... g Fats: ..... g	....

DAILY MACROS	Net Carbs: ..... g Proteins: ..... g Fats: ..... g

Notes:

DAY 31	Date:	Mood Check: ☺ ☺ 😐 ☹ 😖

BREAKFAST	LUNCH	Water:
		🥤🥤🥤🥤🥤 🥤🥤🥤🥤🥤
		Sleep (Hours):
Net Carbs: ..... g Proteins: ..... g Fats: ..... g	Net Carbs: ..... g Proteins: ..... g Fats: ..... g	....

DINNER	SNACKS	Exercise Type:
		....
		Exercise (Minutes):
Net Carbs: ..... g Proteins: ..... g Fats: ..... g	Net Carbs: ..... g Proteins: ..... g Fats: ..... g	....

DAILY MACROS	Net Carbs: ..... g Proteins: ..... g Fats: ..... g

Notes:

DAY 32

Date: ....

Mood Check: 😀 🙂 😐 🙁 😣

BREAKFAST

LUNCH

Water:
🥛🥛🥛🥛🥛
🥛🥛🥛🥛🥛

Sleep (Hours):

Net Carbs: ...... g Proteins: ...... g Fats: ...... g | Net Carbs: ...... g Proteins: ...... g Fats: ...... g | ....

DINNER

SNACKS

Exercise Type:

....

Exercise (Minutes):

Net Carbs: ...... g Proteins: ...... g Fats: ...... g | Net Carbs: ...... g Proteins: ...... g Fats: ...... g

....

DAILY MACROS Net Carbs: ...... g Proteins: ...... g Fats: ...... g

Notes:

DAY 33

Date: ....

Mood Check: 😀 🙂 😐 🙁 😣

BREAKFAST

LUNCH

Water:
🥛🥛🥛🥛🥛
🥛🥛🥛🥛🥛

Sleep (Hours):

Net Carbs: ...... g Proteins: ...... g Fats: ...... g | Net Carbs: ...... g Proteins: ...... g Fats: ...... g | ....

DINNER

SNACKS

Exercise Type:

....

Exercise (Minutes):

Net Carbs: ...... g Proteins: ...... g Fats: ...... g | Net Carbs: ...... g Proteins: ...... g Fats: ...... g

....

DAILY MACROS Net Carbs: ...... g Proteins: ...... g Fats: ...... g

Notes:

DAY 34 Date: .... Mood Check: 😀 ☺ 😐 🙁 ☹

BREAKFAST	LUNCH	Water:
		🥤🥤🥤🥤🥤 🥤🥤🥤🥤🥤
		Sleep (Hours):
Net Carbs: ...... g Proteins: ...... g Fats: ...... g	Net Carbs: ...... g Proteins: ...... g Fats: ...... g	....
DINNER	SNACKS	Exercise Type:
		....
		Exercise (Minutes):
Net Carbs: ...... g Proteins: ...... g Fats: ...... g	Net Carbs: ...... g Proteins: ...... g Fats: ...... g	....
DAILY MACROS Net Carbs: .... g Proteins: .... g Fats: .... g		

Notes:

DAY 35 Date: .... Mood Check: 😀 ☺ 😐 🙁 ☹

BREAKFAST	LUNCH	Water:
		🥤🥤🥤🥤🥤 🥤🥤🥤🥤🥤
		Sleep (Hours):
Net Carbs: ...... g Proteins: ...... g Fats: ...... g	Net Carbs: ...... g Proteins: ...... g Fats: ...... g	....
DINNER	SNACKS	Exercise Type:
		....
		Exercise (Minutes):
Net Carbs: ...... g Proteins: ...... g Fats: ...... g	Net Carbs: ...... g Proteins: ...... g Fats: ...... g	....
DAILY MACROS Net Carbs: .... g Proteins: .... g Fats: .... g		

Notes:

WEEKLY INTENTIONS

What are you excited for this week?

....

....

....

....

What is something you'd like to work on this week? ....

....

....

....

Carbs: .... %
Proteins: .... %
Fats: .... %

DAY 36	Date:	Mood Check: 😀 🙂 😐 🙁 😣

BREAKFAST	LUNCH	Water:
		🥛🥛🥛🥛🥛 🥛🥛🥛🥛🥛
		Sleep (Hours):
Net Carbs: ...... g Proteins: ...... g Fats: ...... g	Net Carbs: ...... g Proteins: ...... g Fats: ...... g	....

DINNER	SNACKS	Exercise Type:
		....
		Exercise (Minutes):
Net Carbs: ...... g Proteins: ...... g Fats: ...... g	Net Carbs: ...... g Proteins: ...... g Fats: ...... g	....

DAILY MACROS	Net Carbs: .... g Proteins: .... g Fats: .... g

Notes:

DAY 37   Date: ....   Mood Check: 😊 🙂 😐 🙁 😣

BREAKFAST	LUNCH	Water:
		🥛🥛🥛🥛🥛 🥛🥛🥛🥛🥛
		Sleep (Hours):
Net Carbs: ...... g Proteins: ...... g Fats: ...... g	Net Carbs: ...... g Proteins: ...... g Fats: ...... g	....
DINNER	**SNACKS**	Exercise Type:
		....
		Exercise (Minutes):
Net Carbs: ...... g Proteins: ...... g Fats: ...... g	Net Carbs: ...... g Proteins: ...... g Fats: ...... g	....
DAILY MACROS Net Carbs: .... g Proteins: .... g Fats: .... g		

Notes:

DAY 38   Date: ....   Mood Check: 😊 🙂 😐 🙁 😣

BREAKFAST	LUNCH	Water:
		🥛🥛🥛🥛🥛 🥛🥛🥛🥛🥛
		Sleep (Hours):
Net Carbs: ...... g Proteins: ...... g Fats: ...... g	Net Carbs: ...... g Proteins: ...... g Fats: ...... g	....
DINNER	**SNACKS**	Exercise Type:
		....
		Exercise (Minutes):
Net Carbs: ...... g Proteins: ...... g Fats: ...... g	Net Carbs: ...... g Proteins: ...... g Fats: ...... g	....
DAILY MACROS Net Carbs: .... g Proteins: .... g Fats: .... g		

Notes:

DAY 39

Date: .... Mood Check: 😃 🙂 😐 🙁 😣

BREAKFAST	LUNCH	Water:
		🥛🥛🥛🥛🥛
		🥛🥛🥛🥛🥛
		Sleep (Hours):
Net Carbs: ...... g Proteins: ...... g Fats: ...... g	Net Carbs: ...... g Proteins: ...... g Fats: ...... g	....
DINNER	**SNACKS**	Exercise Type:
		....
		Exercise (Minutes):
Net Carbs: ...... g Proteins: ...... g Fats: ...... g	Net Carbs: ...... g Proteins: ...... g Fats: ...... g	....

DAILY MACROS   Net Carbs: .... g   Proteins: .... g   Fats: .... g

Notes:

DAY 40

Date: .... Mood Check: 😃 🙂 😐 🙁 😣

BREAKFAST	LUNCH	Water:
		🥛🥛🥛🥛🥛
		🥛🥛🥛🥛🥛
		Sleep (Hours):
Net Carbs: ...... g Proteins: ...... g Fats: ...... g	Net Carbs: ...... g Proteins: ...... g Fats: ...... g	....
DINNER	**SNACKS**	Exercise Type:
		....
		Exercise (Minutes):
Net Carbs: ...... g Proteins: ...... g Fats: ...... g	Net Carbs: ...... g Proteins: ...... g Fats: ...... g	....

DAILY MACROS   Net Carbs: .... g   Proteins: .... g   Fats: .... g

Notes:

DAY 41   Date: ....   Mood Check: 😀 🙂 😐 🙁 😫

BREAKFAST	LUNCH	Water:
		🥛🥛🥛🥛🥛 🥛🥛🥛🥛🥛
		Sleep (Hours):
Net Carbs: ...... g Proteins: ...... g Fats: ...... g	Net Carbs: ...... g Proteins: ...... g Fats: ...... g	....
DINNER	SNACKS	Exercise Type:
		....
		Exercise (Minutes):
Net Carbs: ...... g Proteins: ...... g Fats: ...... g	Net Carbs: ...... g Proteins: ...... g Fats: ...... g	....
DAILY MACROS Net Carbs: ...... g Proteins: ...... g Fats: ...... g		

Notes:

DAY 42   Date: ....   Mood Check: 😀 🙂 😐 🙁 😫

BREAKFAST	LUNCH	Water:
		🥛🥛🥛🥛🥛 🥛🥛🥛🥛🥛
		Sleep (Hours):
Net Carbs: ...... g Proteins: ...... g Fats: ...... g	Net Carbs: ...... g Proteins: ...... g Fats: ...... g	....
DINNER	SNACKS	Exercise Type:
		....
		Exercise (Minutes):
Net Carbs: ...... g Proteins: ...... g Fats: ...... g	Net Carbs: ...... g Proteins: ...... g Fats: ...... g	....
DAILY MACROS Net Carbs: ...... g Proteins: ...... g Fats: ...... g		

Notes:

WEEKLY INTENTIONS

What are you excited for this week?

Carbs: .... %
Proteins: .... %
Fats: .... %

....

....

....

....

What is something you'd like to work on this week? ....

....

....

....

DAY 43 Date: .... Mood Check: 😃 😊 😐 😟 😦

BREAKFAST	LUNCH	Water:
		🥛🥛🥛🥛🥛
		🥛🥛🥛🥛🥛
		Sleep (Hours):
Net Carbs: ...... g Proteins: ...... g Fats: ...... g	Net Carbs: ...... g Proteins: ...... g Fats: ...... g	....
DINNER	**SNACKS**	Exercise Type:
		....
		Exercise (Minutes):
Net Carbs: ...... g Proteins: ...... g Fats: ...... g	Net Carbs: ...... g Proteins: ...... g Fats: ...... g	....

DAILY MACROS   Net Carbs: .... g   Proteins: .... g   Fats: .... g

Notes:

DAY 44 Date: .... Mood Check: 😀 🙂 😐 🙁 😫

BREAKFAST	LUNCH	Water:
		🥤🥤🥤🥤🥤 🥤🥤🥤🥤🥤
		Sleep (Hours):
Net Carbs: ...... g Proteins: ...... g Fats: ...... g	Net Carbs: ...... g Proteins: ...... g Fats: ...... g	....
DINNER	SNACKS	Exercise Type:
		....
		Exercise (Minutes):
Net Carbs: ...... g Proteins: ...... g Fats: ...... g	Net Carbs: ...... g Proteins: ...... g Fats: ...... g	....
DAILY MACROS Net Carbs: .... g Proteins: .... g Fats: .... g		

Notes:

DAY 45 Date: .... Mood Check: 😀 🙂 😐 🙁 😫

BREAKFAST	LUNCH	Water:
		🥤🥤🥤🥤🥤 🥤🥤🥤🥤🥤
		Sleep (Hours):
Net Carbs: ...... g Proteins: ...... g Fats: ...... g	Net Carbs: ...... g Proteins: ...... g Fats: ...... g	....
DINNER	SNACKS	Exercise Type:
		....
		Exercise (Minutes):
Net Carbs: ...... g Proteins: ...... g Fats: ...... g	Net Carbs: ...... g Proteins: ...... g Fats: ...... g	....
DAILY MACROS Net Carbs: .... g Proteins: .... g Fats: .... g		

Notes:

DAY 46 | Date: .... Mood Check: 😃 😊 😐 🙁 😫

BREAKFAST	LUNCH	Water:
		🥛🥛🥛🥛🥛 🥛🥛🥛🥛🥛
		Sleep (Hours):
Net Carbs: ...... g Proteins: ...... g Fats: ...... g	Net Carbs: ...... g Proteins: ...... g Fats: ...... g	....
DINNER	**SNACKS**	Exercise Type: .... Exercise (Minutes):
Net Carbs: ...... g Proteins: ...... g Fats: ...... g	Net Carbs: ...... g Proteins: ...... g Fats: ...... g	....
DAILY MACROS Net Carbs: ...... g Proteins: ...... g Fats: ...... g		

Notes:

DAY 47 | Date: .... Mood Check: 😃 😊 😐 🙁 😫

BREAKFAST	LUNCH	Water:
		🥛🥛🥛🥛🥛 🥛🥛🥛🥛🥛
		Sleep (Hours):
Net Carbs: ...... g Proteins: ...... g Fats: ...... g	Net Carbs: ...... g Proteins: ...... g Fats: ...... g	....
DINNER	**SNACKS**	Exercise Type: .... Exercise (Minutes):
Net Carbs: ...... g Proteins: ...... g Fats: ...... g	Net Carbs: ...... g Proteins: ...... g Fats: ...... g	....
DAILY MACROS Net Carbs: ...... g Proteins: ...... g Fats: ...... g		

Notes:

DAY 48	Date:	Mood Check: 😀 🙂 😐 🙁 😣

BREAKFAST	**LUNCH**	Water: 🥛🥛🥛🥛🥛 🥛🥛🥛🥛🥛
		Sleep (Hours):
Net Carbs: ...... g Proteins: ...... g Fats: ...... g	Net Carbs: ...... g Proteins: ...... g Fats: ...... g	....

DINNER	**SNACKS**	Exercise Type: .... Exercise (Minutes):
Net Carbs: ...... g Proteins: ...... g Fats: ...... g	Net Carbs: ...... g Proteins: ...... g Fats: ...... g	....

DAILY MACROS	Net Carbs: ...... g Proteins: ...... g Fats: ...... g

Notes:

DAY 49	Date:	Mood Check: 😀 🙂 😐 🙁 😣

BREAKFAST	**LUNCH**	Water: 🥛🥛🥛🥛🥛 🥛🥛🥛🥛🥛
		Sleep (Hours):
Net Carbs: ...... g Proteins: ...... g Fats: ...... g	Net Carbs: ...... g Proteins: ...... g Fats: ...... g	....

DINNER	**SNACKS**	Exercise Type: .... Exercise (Minutes):
Net Carbs: ...... g Proteins: ...... g Fats: ...... g	Net Carbs: ...... g Proteins: ...... g Fats: ...... g	....

DAILY MACROS	Net Carbs: ...... g Proteins: ...... g Fats: ...... g

Notes:

WEEKLY INTENTIONS

What are you excited for this week?

....

....

....

What is something you'd like to work on this week? ....

....

....

....

Carbs: .... %
Proteins: .... %
Fats: .... %

DAY 50   Date: ....   Mood Check: 😀 😊 😐 🙁 ☹️

BREAKFAST	LUNCH	Water:
		🥛🥛🥛🥛🥛 🥛🥛🥛🥛🥛
		Sleep (Hours):
Net Carbs: ...... g Proteins: ...... g Fats: ...... g	Net Carbs: ...... g Proteins: ...... g Fats: ...... g	....
DINNER	**SNACKS**	Exercise Type:
		....
		Exercise (Minutes):
Net Carbs: ...... g Proteins: ...... g Fats: ...... g	Net Carbs: ...... g Proteins: ...... g Fats: ...... g	....
DAILY MACROS Net Carbs: ...... g Proteins: ...... g Fats: ...... g		

Notes:

DAY 51   Date: ....   Mood Check: 😄 😊 😐 🙁 😞

BREAKFAST	LUNCH	Water:
		🥤🥤🥤🥤🥤 🥤🥤🥤🥤🥤
		Sleep (Hours):
Net Carbs: ...... g Proteins: ...... g Fats: ...... g	Net Carbs: ...... g Proteins: ...... g Fats: ...... g	....
DINNER	SNACKS	Exercise Type:
		....
		Exercise (Minutes):
Net Carbs: ...... g Proteins: ...... g Fats: ...... g	Net Carbs: ...... g Proteins: ...... g Fats: ...... g	....

DAILY MACROS   Net Carbs: .... g   Proteins: .... g   Fats: .... g

Notes:

DAY 52   Date: ....   Mood Check: 😄 😊 😐 🙁 😞

BREAKFAST	LUNCH	Water:
		🥤🥤🥤🥤🥤 🥤🥤🥤🥤🥤
		Sleep (Hours):
Net Carbs: ...... g Proteins: ...... g Fats: ...... g	Net Carbs: ...... g Proteins: ...... g Fats: ...... g	....
DINNER	SNACKS	Exercise Type:
		....
		Exercise (Minutes):
Net Carbs: ...... g Proteins: ...... g Fats: ...... g	Net Carbs: ...... g Proteins: ...... g Fats: ...... g	....

DAILY MACROS   Net Carbs: .... g   Proteins: .... g   Fats: .... g

Notes:

DAY 53 Date: .... Mood Check: 😀 😊 😐 😕 😣

BREAKFAST	LUNCH	Water:
		🥛🥛🥛🥛🥛 🥛🥛🥛🥛🥛
		Sleep (Hours):
Net Carbs: ...... g Proteins: ...... g Fats: ...... g	Net Carbs: ...... g Proteins: ...... g Fats: ...... g	....

DINNER	SNACKS	Exercise Type:
		....
		Exercise (Minutes):
Net Carbs: ...... g Proteins: ...... g Fats: ...... g	Net Carbs: ...... g Proteins: ...... g Fats: ...... g	....

DAILY MACROS Net Carbs: ...... g Proteins: ...... g Fats: ...... g

Notes:

DAY 54 Date: .... Mood Check: 😀 😊 😐 😕 😣

BREAKFAST	LUNCH	Water:
		🥛🥛🥛🥛🥛 🥛🥛🥛🥛🥛
		Sleep (Hours):
Net Carbs: ...... g Proteins: ...... g Fats: ...... g	Net Carbs: ...... g Proteins: ...... g Fats: ...... g	....

DINNER	SNACKS	Exercise Type:
		....
		Exercise (Minutes):
Net Carbs: ...... g Proteins: ...... g Fats: ...... g	Net Carbs: ...... g Proteins: ...... g Fats: ...... g	....

DAILY MACROS Net Carbs: ...... g Proteins: ...... g Fats: ...... g

Notes:

| DAY 55 | Date: .... | Mood Check: ☺ ☺ ☺ ☹ ☹ |

DAY 55   Date: ....   Mood Check: ☺ ☺ ☺ ☹ ☹

BREAKFAST	LUNCH	Water:
		🥤🥤🥤🥤 🥤🥤🥤🥤
		Sleep (Hours):
Net Carbs: ...... g Proteins: ...... g Fats: ...... g	Net Carbs: ...... g Proteins: ...... g Fats: ...... g	....
DINNER	**SNACKS**	Exercise Type:
		....
		Exercise (Minutes):
Net Carbs: ...... g Proteins: ...... g Fats: ...... g	Net Carbs: ...... g Proteins: ...... g Fats: ...... g	
DAILY MACROS Net Carbs: ...... g Proteins: ...... g Fats: ...... g		....

Notes:

DAY 56   Date: ....   Mood Check: ☺ ☺ ☺ ☹ ☹

BREAKFAST	LUNCH	Water:
		🥤🥤🥤🥤 🥤🥤🥤🥤
		Sleep (Hours):
Net Carbs: ...... g Proteins: ...... g Fats: ...... g	Net Carbs: ...... g Proteins: ...... g Fats: ...... g	....
DINNER	**SNACKS**	Exercise Type:
		....
		Exercise (Minutes):
Net Carbs: ...... g Proteins: ...... g Fats: ...... g	Net Carbs: ...... g Proteins: ...... g Fats: ...... g	
DAILY MACROS Net Carbs: ...... g Proteins: ...... g Fats: ...... g		....

Notes:

MEASUREMENT	CURRENT	MONTH CHANGE
WEIGHT (LBS)		
UPPER ARMS (IN)		
CHEST (IN)		
WAIST (IN)		
HIPS (IN)		
THIGHS (IN)		
CALVES (IN)		

CHECKING IN

Congratulations on making it this far! What are you most proud of from the past 4 weeks?

What was your biggest challenge over the past 4 weeks?

....

....

....

....

....

....

What are some goals you would like to work toward over the
next 4 weeks?

....

....

....

....

....

....

Reflect on your mood over the past month—did you notice
differences related to your eating habits?

....

....

....

....

....

WEEKLY INTENTIONS

What are you excited for this week?

Carbs: .... %
Proteins: .... %
Fats: .... %

....

....

....

What is something you'd like to work on this week? ....

....

....

....

DAY 57	Date:	Mood Check: 😃 😊 😐 🙁 ☹️
BREAKFAST	**LUNCH**	Water: 🥛🥛🥛🥛🥛 🥛🥛🥛🥛🥛
		Sleep (Hours):
Net Carbs: ...... g Proteins: ...... g Fats: ...... g	Net Carbs: ...... g Proteins: ...... g Fats: ...... g	
DINNER	**SNACKS**	Exercise Type:
		Exercise (Minutes):
Net Carbs: ...... g Proteins: ...... g Fats: ...... g	Net Carbs: ...... g Proteins: ...... g Fats: ...... g	
DAILY MACROS	Net Carbs: ...... g Proteins: ...... g Fats: ...... g	

Notes:

DAY 58   Date: .... Mood Check: 😀 😊 😐 😕 😣

BREAKFAST	LUNCH	Water: 🥛🥛🥛🥛 🥛🥛🥛🥛
		Sleep (Hours):
Net Carbs: ...... g Proteins: ...... g Fats: ...... g	Net Carbs: ...... g Proteins: ...... g Fats: ...... g	....
DINNER	SNACKS	Exercise Type: .... Exercise (Minutes):
Net Carbs: ...... g Proteins: ...... g Fats: ...... g	Net Carbs: ...... g Proteins: ...... g Fats: ...... g	....

DAILY MACROS   Net Carbs: ...... g   Proteins: ...... g   Fats: ...... g

Notes:

DAY 59   Date: .... Mood Check: 😀 😊 😐 😕 😣

BREAKFAST	LUNCH	Water: 🥛🥛🥛🥛 🥛🥛🥛🥛
		Sleep (Hours):
Net Carbs: ...... g Proteins: ...... g Fats: ...... g	Net Carbs: ...... g Proteins: ...... g Fats: ...... g	....
DINNER	SNACKS	Exercise Type: .... Exercise (Minutes):
Net Carbs: ...... g Proteins: ...... g Fats: ...... g	Net Carbs: ...... g Proteins: ...... g Fats: ...... g	....

DAILY MACROS   Net Carbs: ...... g   Proteins: ...... g   Fats: ...... g

Notes:

DAY 60 Date: .... Mood Check: 😀 😊 😐 😕 😣

BREAKFAST	LUNCH	Water:
		🥛🥛🥛🥛🥛 🥛🥛🥛🥛🥛
		Sleep (Hours):
Net Carbs: ...... g Proteins: ...... g Fats: ...... g	Net Carbs: ...... g Proteins: ...... g Fats: ...... g	....
DINNER	SNACKS	Exercise Type:
		....
		Exercise (Minutes):
Net Carbs: ...... g Proteins: ...... g Fats: ...... g	Net Carbs: ...... g Proteins: ...... g Fats: ...... g	....
DAILY MACROS	Net Carbs: ...... g Proteins: ...... g Fats: ...... g	

Notes:

DAY 61 Date: .... Mood Check: 😀 😊 😐 😕 😣

BREAKFAST	LUNCH	Water:
		🥛🥛🥛🥛🥛 🥛🥛🥛🥛🥛
		Sleep (Hours):
Net Carbs: ...... g Proteins: ...... g Fats: ...... g	Net Carbs: ...... g Proteins: ...... g Fats: ...... g	....
DINNER	SNACKS	Exercise Type:
		....
		Exercise (Minutes):
Net Carbs: ...... g Proteins: ...... g Fats: ...... g	Net Carbs: ...... g Proteins: ...... g Fats: ...... g	....
DAILY MACROS	Net Carbs: ...... g Proteins: ...... g Fats: ...... g	

Notes:

DAY 62   Date: ....   Mood Check: 😃 😊 😐 😟 😣

BREAKFAST	LUNCH	Water:
		🥤🥤🥤🥤🥤 🥤🥤🥤🥤🥤
		Sleep (Hours):
Net Carbs: ...... g Proteins: ...... g Fats: ...... g	Net Carbs: ...... g Proteins: ...... g Fats: ...... g	....
DINNER	SNACKS	Exercise Type:
		....
		Exercise (Minutes):
Net Carbs: ...... g Proteins: ...... g Fats: ...... g	Net Carbs: ...... g Proteins: ...... g Fats: ...... g	....

DAILY MACROS	Net Carbs: ...... g Proteins: ...... g Fats: ...... g

Notes:

DAY 63   Date: ....   Mood Check: 😃 😊 😐 😟 😣

BREAKFAST	LUNCH	Water:
		🥤🥤🥤🥤🥤 🥤🥤🥤🥤🥤
		Sleep (Hours):
Net Carbs: ...... g Proteins: ...... g Fats: ...... g	Net Carbs: ...... g Proteins: ...... g Fats: ...... g	....
DINNER	SNACKS	Exercise Type:
		....
		Exercise (Minutes):
Net Carbs: ...... g Proteins: ...... g Fats: ...... g	Net Carbs: ...... g Proteins: ...... g Fats: ...... g	....

DAILY MACROS	Net Carbs: ...... g Proteins: ...... g Fats: ...... g

Notes:

WEEKLY INTENTIONS

What are you excited for this week?

....

....

....

....

Carbs: .... %
Proteins: .... %
Fats: .... %

What is something you'd like to work on this week? ....

....

....

....

DAY 64	Date:	Mood Check: 😃 😊 😐 🙁 😣	
BREAKFAST	**LUNCH**	Water: 🥤🥤🥤🥤🥤 🥤🥤🥤🥤🥤	
		Sleep (Hours):	
Net Carbs: ...... g Proteins: ...... g Fats: ...... g	Net Carbs: ...... g Proteins: ...... g Fats: ...... g	....	
DINNER	**SNACKS**	Exercise Type: .... Exercise (Minutes):	
Net Carbs: ...... g Proteins: ...... g Fats: ...... g	Net Carbs: ...... g Proteins: ...... g Fats: ...... g	....	
DAILY MACROS	Net Carbs: .... g Proteins: .... g Fats: .... g		

Notes:

DAY 65 Date: .... Mood Check: 😃 😊 😐 🙁 😞

BREAKFAST	LUNCH	Water:
		🥛🥛🥛🥛🥛 🥛🥛🥛🥛🥛
		Sleep (Hours):
Net Carbs: ...... g Proteins: ...... g Fats: ...... g	Net Carbs: ...... g Proteins: ...... g Fats: ...... g	....
DINNER	SNACKS	Exercise Type:
		....
		Exercise (Minutes):
Net Carbs: ...... g Proteins: ...... g Fats: ...... g	Net Carbs: ...... g Proteins: ...... g Fats: ...... g	....
DAILY MACROS Net Carbs: ...... g Proteins: ...... g Fats: ...... g		

Notes:

DAY 66 Date: .... Mood Check: 😃 😊 😐 🙁 😞

BREAKFAST	LUNCH	Water:
		🥛🥛🥛🥛🥛 🥛🥛🥛🥛🥛
		Sleep (Hours):
Net Carbs: ...... g Proteins: ...... g Fats: ...... g	Net Carbs: ...... g Proteins: ...... g Fats: ...... g	....
DINNER	SNACKS	Exercise Type:
		....
		Exercise (Minutes):
Net Carbs: ...... g Proteins: ...... g Fats: ...... g	Net Carbs: ...... g Proteins: ...... g Fats: ...... g	....
DAILY MACROS Net Carbs: ...... g Proteins: ...... g Fats: ...... g		

Notes:

DAY 67 Date: .... Mood Check: 😃 😊 😐 😟 😣

BREAKFAST	LUNCH	Water:

Sleep (Hours):

Net Carbs: ...... g Proteins: ...... g Fats: ...... g | Net Carbs: ...... g Proteins: ...... g Fats: ...... g | ....

DINNER	SNACKS	Exercise Type:

Exercise (Minutes):

Net Carbs: ...... g Proteins: ...... g Fats: ...... g | Net Carbs: ...... g Proteins: ...... g Fats: ...... g

DAILY MACROS   Net Carbs: ...... g   Proteins: ...... g   Fats: ...... g

Notes:

DAY 68 Date: .... Mood Check: 😃 😊 😐 😟 😣

BREAKFAST	LUNCH	Water:

Sleep (Hours):

Net Carbs: ...... g Proteins: ...... g Fats: ...... g | Net Carbs: ...... g Proteins: ...... g Fats: ...... g | ....

DINNER	SNACKS	Exercise Type:

Exercise (Minutes):

Net Carbs: ...... g Proteins: ...... g Fats: ...... g | Net Carbs: ...... g Proteins: ...... g Fats: ...... g

DAILY MACROS   Net Carbs: ...... g   Proteins: ...... g   Fats: ...... g

Notes:

DAY 69 Date: .... Mood Check: 😀 🙂 😐 🙁 😣

BREAKFAST	LUNCH	Water:
		🥤🥤🥤🥤🥤 🥤🥤🥤🥤🥤
		Sleep (Hours):
Net Carbs: ...... g Proteins: ...... g Fats: ...... g	Net Carbs: ...... g Proteins: ...... g Fats: ...... g	....
DINNER	SNACKS	Exercise Type:
		....
		Exercise (Minutes):
Net Carbs: ...... g Proteins: ...... g Fats: ...... g	Net Carbs: ...... g Proteins: ...... g Fats: ...... g	....
DAILY MACROS Net Carbs: ...... g Proteins: ...... g Fats: ...... g		

Notes:

DAY 70 Date: .... Mood Check: 😀 🙂 😐 🙁 😣

BREAKFAST	LUNCH	Water:
		🥤🥤🥤🥤🥤 🥤🥤🥤🥤🥤
		Sleep (Hours):
Net Carbs: ...... g Proteins: ...... g Fats: ...... g	Net Carbs: ...... g Proteins: ...... g Fats: ...... g	....
DINNER	SNACKS	Exercise Type:
		....
		Exercise (Minutes):
Net Carbs: ...... g Proteins: ...... g Fats: ...... g	Net Carbs: ...... g Proteins: ...... g Fats: ...... g	....
DAILY MACROS Net Carbs: ...... g Proteins: ...... g Fats: ...... g		

Notes:

WEEKLY INTENTIONS

What are you excited for this week?

....

....

What is something you'd like to work on this week? ....

....

....

....

DAY 71	Date:	Mood Check: 😄 🙂 😐 🙁 😣

BREAKFAST	LUNCH	Water:
		🥛🥛🥛🥛🥛 🥛🥛🥛🥛🥛
		Sleep (Hours):
Net Carbs: ......g Proteins: ......g Fats: ......g	Net Carbs: ......g Proteins: ......g Fats: ......g	....
DINNER	SNACKS	Exercise Type: .... Exercise (Minutes):
Net Carbs: ......g Proteins: ......g Fats: ......g	Net Carbs: ......g Proteins: ......g Fats: ......g	....
DAILY MACROS Net Carbs: ......g Proteins: ......g Fats: ......g		

Notes:

DAY 72	Date:	Mood Check: 😀 😊 😐 😕 😣
BREAKFAST	**LUNCH**	Water: 🥛🥛🥛🥛🥛 🥛🥛🥛🥛🥛
		Sleep (Hours):
Net Carbs: ...... g Proteins: ...... g Fats: ...... g	Net Carbs: ...... g Proteins: ...... g Fats: ...... g	....
DINNER	**SNACKS**	Exercise Type: ....
		Exercise (Minutes):
Net Carbs: ...... g Proteins: ...... g Fats: ...... g	Net Carbs: ...... g Proteins: ...... g Fats: ...... g	....
DAILY MACROS Net Carbs: ...... g Proteins: ...... g Fats: ...... g		

Notes:

DAY 73	Date:	Mood Check: 😀 😊 😐 😕 😣
BREAKFAST	**LUNCH**	Water: 🥛🥛🥛🥛🥛 🥛🥛🥛🥛🥛
		Sleep (Hours):
Net Carbs: ...... g Proteins: ...... g Fats: ...... g	Net Carbs: ...... g Proteins: ...... g Fats: ...... g	....
DINNER	**SNACKS**	Exercise Type: ....
		Exercise (Minutes):
Net Carbs: ...... g Proteins: ...... g Fats: ...... g	Net Carbs: ...... g Proteins: ...... g Fats: ...... g	....
DAILY MACROS Net Carbs: ...... g Proteins: ...... g Fats: ...... g		

Notes:

DAY 74 Date: .... Mood Check: 😃 😊 😐 🙁 😣

BREAKFAST	LUNCH	Water:
		🥛🥛🥛🥛🥛 🥛🥛🥛🥛🥛
		Sleep (Hours):
Net Carbs: ...... g Proteins: ...... g Fats: ...... g	Net Carbs: ...... g Proteins: ...... g Fats: ...... g	....
DINNER	**SNACKS**	Exercise Type: .... Exercise (Minutes):
Net Carbs: ...... g Proteins: ...... g Fats: ...... g	Net Carbs: ...... g Proteins: ...... g Fats: ...... g	....

DAILY MACROS   Net Carbs: ...... g   Proteins: ...... g   Fats: ...... g

Notes:

DAY 75 Date: .... Mood Check: 😃 😊 😐 🙁 😣

BREAKFAST	LUNCH	Water:
		🥛🥛🥛🥛🥛 🥛🥛🥛🥛🥛
		Sleep (Hours):
Net Carbs: ...... g Proteins: ...... g Fats: ...... g	Net Carbs: ...... g Proteins: ...... g Fats: ...... g	....
DINNER	**SNACKS**	Exercise Type: .... Exercise (Minutes):
Net Carbs: ...... g Proteins: ...... g Fats: ...... g	Net Carbs: ...... g Proteins: ...... g Fats: ...... g	....

DAILY MACROS   Net Carbs: ...... g   Proteins: ...... g   Fats: ...... g

Notes:

DAY 76	Date:	Mood Check: ☺ ☺ ☺ ☹ ☹

BREAKFAST	**LUNCH**	Water:
		🥛🥛🥛🥛🥛 🥛🥛🥛🥛🥛
		Sleep (Hours):
Net Carbs: ...... g Proteins: ...... g Fats: ...... g	Net Carbs: ...... g Proteins: ...... g Fats: ...... g	....
DINNER	**SNACKS**	Exercise Type:
		....
		Exercise (Minutes):
Net Carbs: ...... g Proteins: ...... g Fats: ...... g	Net Carbs: ...... g Proteins: ...... g Fats: ...... g	....
DAILY MACROS Net Carbs: ...... g Proteins: ...... g Fats: ...... g		

Notes:

DAY 77	Date:	Mood Check: ☺ ☺ ☺ ☹ ☹

BREAKFAST	**LUNCH**	Water:
		🥛🥛🥛🥛🥛 🥛🥛🥛🥛🥛
		Sleep (Hours):
Net Carbs: ...... g Proteins: ...... g Fats: ...... g	Net Carbs: ...... g Proteins: ...... g Fats: ...... g	....
DINNER	**SNACKS**	Exercise Type:
		....
		Exercise (Minutes):
Net Carbs: ...... g Proteins: ...... g Fats: ...... g	Net Carbs: ...... g Proteins: ...... g Fats: ...... g	....
DAILY MACROS Net Carbs: ...... g Proteins: ...... g Fats: ...... g		

Notes:

WEEKLY INTENTIONS

What are you excited for this week?

....

....

....

....

What is something you'd like to work on this week? ....

....

....

....

DAY 78	Date:	Mood Check: 😊 🙂 😐 🙁 ☹️

BREAKFAST	LUNCH	Water:
		🥤🥤🥤🥤🥤 🥤🥤🥤🥤🥤
		Sleep (Hours):
Net Carbs: ...... g Proteins: ...... g Fats: ...... g	Net Carbs: ...... g Proteins: ...... g Fats: ...... g	....
DINNER	**SNACKS**	Exercise Type:
		....
		Exercise (Minutes):
Net Carbs: ...... g Proteins: ...... g Fats: ...... g	Net Carbs: ...... g Proteins: ...... g Fats: ...... g	....

DAILY MACROS	Net Carbs: ...... g Proteins: ...... g Fats: ...... g

Notes:

DAY 79 Date: .... Mood Check: 😃 🙂 😐 🙁 😣

BREAKFAST	LUNCH	Water: 🥤🥤🥤🥤🥤 🥤🥤🥤🥤🥤
		Sleep (Hours):
Net Carbs: ...... g Proteins: ...... g Fats: ...... g	Net Carbs: ...... g Proteins: ...... g Fats: ...... g	....
DINNER	SNACKS	Exercise Type: .... Exercise (Minutes):
Net Carbs: ...... g Proteins: ...... g Fats: ...... g	Net Carbs: ...... g Proteins: ...... g Fats: ...... g	....
DAILY MACROS Net Carbs: ...... g Proteins: ...... g Fats: ...... g		

Notes:

DAY 80 Date: .... Mood Check: 😃 🙂 😐 🙁 😣

BREAKFAST	LUNCH	Water: 🥤🥤🥤🥤🥤 🥤🥤🥤🥤🥤
		Sleep (Hours):
Net Carbs: ...... g Proteins: ...... g Fats: ...... g	Net Carbs: ...... g Proteins: ...... g Fats: ...... g	....
DINNER	SNACKS	Exercise Type: .... Exercise (Minutes):
Net Carbs: ...... g Proteins: ...... g Fats: ...... g	Net Carbs: ...... g Proteins: ...... g Fats: ...... g	....
DAILY MACROS Net Carbs: ...... g Proteins: ...... g Fats: ...... g		

Notes:

DAY 81 Date: .... Mood Check: 😊 😊 😐 🙁 ☹️

BREAKFAST

LUNCH

Water:

Net Carbs: ...... g Proteins: ...... g Fats: ...... g

Net Carbs: ...... g Proteins: ...... g Fats: ...... g

Sleep (Hours):

....

DINNER

SNACKS

Exercise Type:

....

Exercise (Minutes):

Net Carbs: ...... g Proteins: ...... g Fats: ...... g

Net Carbs: ...... g Proteins: ...... g Fats: ...... g

....

DAILY MACROS Net Carbs: ...... g Proteins: ...... g Fats: ...... g

Notes:

DAY 82 Date: .... Mood Check: 😊 😊 😐 🙁 ☹️

BREAKFAST

LUNCH

Water:

Net Carbs: ...... g Proteins: ...... g Fats: ...... g

Net Carbs: ...... g Proteins: ...... g Fats: ...... g

Sleep (Hours):

....

DINNER

SNACKS

Exercise Type:

....

Exercise (Minutes):

Net Carbs: ...... g Proteins: ...... g Fats: ...... g

Net Carbs: ...... g Proteins: ...... g Fats: ...... g

....

DAILY MACROS Net Carbs: ...... g Proteins: ...... g Fats: ...... g

Notes:

DAY 83	Date:	Mood Check: 😀 🙂 😐 🙁 😞

BREAKFAST

LUNCH

Water:

🥛🥛🥛🥛🥛
🥛🥛🥛🥛🥛

Net Carbs: ...... g Proteins: ...... g Fats: ...... g

Net Carbs: ...... g Proteins: ...... g Fats: ...... g

Sleep (Hours):

....

DINNER

SNACKS

Exercise Type:

....

Exercise (Minutes):

Net Carbs: ...... g Proteins: ...... g Fats: ...... g

Net Carbs: ...... g Proteins: ...... g Fats: ...... g

....

DAILY MACROS   Net Carbs: .... g   Proteins: .... g   Fats: .... g

Notes:

DAY 84	Date:	Mood Check: 😀 🙂 😐 🙁 😞

BREAKFAST

LUNCH

Water:

🥛🥛🥛🥛🥛
🥛🥛🥛🥛🥛

Net Carbs: ...... g Proteins: ...... g Fats: ...... g

Net Carbs: ...... g Proteins: ...... g Fats: ...... g

Sleep (Hours):

....

DINNER

SNACKS

Exercise Type:

....

Exercise (Minutes):

Net Carbs: ...... g Proteins: ...... g Fats: ...... g

Net Carbs: ...... g Proteins: ...... g Fats: ...... g

....

DAILY MACROS   Net Carbs: .... g   Proteins: .... g   Fats: .... g

Notes:

MEASUREMENT	CURRENT	MONTH CHANGE
WEIGHT (LBS)		
UPPER ARMS (IN)		
CHEST (IN)		
WAIST (IN)		
HIPS (IN)		
THIGHS (IN)		
CALVES (IN)		

CHECKING IN

Congratulations on making it this far! What are you most proud of from the past 4 weeks?

....

....

....

....

....

What was your biggest challenge over the past 4 weeks?

....

....

....

....

....

....

What are some goals you would like to work toward over the
next 4 weeks?

....

....

....

....

....

Reflect on your mood over the past month—did you notice
differences related to your eating habits?

....

....

....

....

....

WEEKLY INTENTIONS

What are you excited for this week?

....

....

....

What is something you'd like to work on this week? ....

....

....

....

Carbs: .... %
Proteins: .... %
Fats: .... %

DAY 85 | Date: .... Mood Check: 😀 🙂 😐 🙁 😣

BREAKFAST	LUNCH	Water:
		🥤🥤🥤🥤🥤 🥤🥤🥤🥤🥤
		Sleep (Hours):
Net Carbs: ...... g Proteins: ...... g Fats: ...... g	Net Carbs: ...... g Proteins: ...... g Fats: ...... g	
DINNER	SNACKS	Exercise Type: .... Exercise (Minutes):
Net Carbs: ...... g Proteins: ...... g Fats: ...... g	Net Carbs: ...... g Proteins: ...... g Fats: ...... g	....

DAILY MACROS | Net Carbs: ...... g Proteins: ...... g Fats: ...... g

Notes:

DAY 86

Date: .... Mood Check: 😃 😊 😐 🙁 ☹️

BREAKFAST

Net Carbs: ...... g Proteins: ...... g Fats: ...... g

LUNCH

Net Carbs: ...... g Proteins: ...... g Fats: ...... g

Water:

Sleep (Hours):

....

DINNER

Net Carbs: ...... g Proteins: ...... g Fats: ...... g

SNACKS

Net Carbs: ...... g Proteins: ...... g Fats: ...... g

Exercise Type:

....

Exercise (Minutes):

....

DAILY MACROS   Net Carbs: ...... g   Proteins: ...... g   Fats: ...... g

Notes:

DAY 87

Date: .... Mood Check: 😃 😊 😐 🙁 ☹️

BREAKFAST

Net Carbs: ...... g Proteins: ...... g Fats: ...... g

LUNCH

Net Carbs: ...... g Proteins: ...... g Fats: ...... g

Water:

Sleep (Hours):

....

DINNER

Net Carbs: ...... g Proteins: ...... g Fats: ...... g

SNACKS

Net Carbs: ...... g Proteins: ...... g Fats: ...... g

Exercise Type:

....

Exercise (Minutes):

....

DAILY MACROS   Net Carbs: ...... g   Proteins: ...... g   Fats: ...... g

Notes:

DAY 88

Date: .... Mood Check: 😃 🙂 😐 🙁 😟

BREAKFAST

Net Carbs: ...... g Proteins: ...... g Fats: ...... g

LUNCH

Net Carbs: ...... g Proteins: ...... g Fats: ...... g

DINNER

Net Carbs: ...... g Proteins: ...... g Fats: ...... g

SNACKS

Net Carbs: ...... g Proteins: ...... g Fats: ...... g

DAILY MACROS   Net Carbs: ...... g   Proteins: ...... g   Fats: ...... g

Water:

Sleep (Hours):
....

Exercise Type:
....

Exercise (Minutes):
....

Notes:

DAY 89

Date: .... Mood Check: 😃 🙂 😐 🙁 😟

BREAKFAST

Net Carbs: ...... g Proteins: ...... g Fats: ...... g

LUNCH

Net Carbs: ...... g Proteins: ...... g Fats: ...... g

DINNER

Net Carbs: ...... g Proteins: ...... g Fats: ...... g

SNACKS

Net Carbs: ...... g Proteins: ...... g Fats: ...... g

DAILY MACROS   Net Carbs: ...... g   Proteins: ...... g   Fats: ...... g

Water:

Sleep (Hours):
....

Exercise Type:
....

Exercise (Minutes):
....

Notes:

DAY 90 Date: .... Mood Check: 😃 😊 😐 🙁 ☹️

BREAKFAST	LUNCH	Water:
		🥤🥤🥤🥤 🥤🥤🥤🥤
		Sleep (Hours):
Net Carbs: ...... g Proteins: ...... g Fats: ...... g	Net Carbs: ...... g Proteins: ...... g Fats: ...... g	....
DINNER	SNACKS	Exercise Type:
		....
		Exercise (Minutes):
Net Carbs: ...... g Proteins: ...... g Fats: ...... g	Net Carbs: ...... g Proteins: ...... g Fats: ...... g	....
DAILY MACROS Net Carbs: ...... g Proteins: ...... g Fats: ...... g		

Notes:

DAY 91 Date: .... Mood Check: 😃 😊 😐 🙁 ☹️

BREAKFAST	LUNCH	Water:
		🥤🥤🥤🥤 🥤🥤🥤🥤
		Sleep (Hours):
Net Carbs: ...... g Proteins: ...... g Fats: ...... g	Net Carbs: ...... g Proteins: ...... g Fats: ...... g	....
DINNER	SNACKS	Exercise Type:
		....
		Exercise (Minutes):
Net Carbs: ...... g Proteins: ...... g Fats: ...... g	Net Carbs: ...... g Proteins: ...... g Fats: ...... g	....
DAILY MACROS Net Carbs: ...... g Proteins: ...... g Fats: ...... g		

Notes:

WEEKLY INTENTIONS

What are you excited for this week?

Carbs: .... %
Proteins: .... %
Fats: .... %

What is something you'd like to work on this week?

DAY 92	Date:	Mood Check: ☺ ☺ ☺ ☹ ☹

BREAKFAST	LUNCH	Water:
		🥤🥤🥤🥤🥤 🥤🥤🥤🥤🥤
		Sleep (Hours):
Net Carbs: ...... g Proteins: ...... g Fats: ...... g	Net Carbs: ...... g Proteins: ...... g Fats: ...... g	....
DINNER	**SNACKS**	Exercise Type:
		....
		Exercise (Minutes):
Net Carbs: ...... g Proteins: ...... g Fats: ...... g	Net Carbs: ...... g Proteins: ...... g Fats: ...... g	....
DAILY MACROS	Net Carbs: ...... g Proteins: ...... g Fats: ...... g	

Notes:

DAY 93

Date: .... Mood Check: 😃 😊 😐 🙁 😞

BREAKFAST

Net Carbs: ...... g Proteins: ...... g Fats: ...... g

LUNCH

Net Carbs: ...... g Proteins: ...... g Fats: ...... g

Water:

Sleep (Hours):

....

DINNER

Net Carbs: ...... g Proteins: ...... g Fats: ...... g

SNACKS

Net Carbs: ...... g Proteins: ...... g Fats: ...... g

Exercise
Type:

....

Exercise
(Minutes):

....

DAILY MACROS   Net Carbs: .... g   Proteins: .... g   Fats: .... g

Notes:

DAY 94

Date: .... Mood Check: 😃 😊 😐 🙁 😞

BREAKFAST

Net Carbs: ...... g Proteins: ...... g Fats: ...... g

LUNCH

Net Carbs: ...... g Proteins: ...... g Fats: ...... g

Water:

Sleep (Hours):

....

DINNER

Net Carbs: ...... g Proteins: ...... g Fats: ...... g

SNACKS

Net Carbs: ...... g Proteins: ...... g Fats: ...... g

Exercise
Type:

....

Exercise
(Minutes):

....

DAILY MACROS   Net Carbs: .... g   Proteins: .... g   Fats: .... g

Notes:

DAY 95 | Date: .... Mood Check: 😃 🙂 😐 🙁 ☹️

BREAKFAST

LUNCH

Water:

🥤🥤🥤🥤
🥤🥤🥤🥤

Net Carbs: ...... g Proteins: ...... g Fats: ...... g

Net Carbs: ...... g Proteins: ...... g Fats: ...... g

Sleep (Hours):

....

DINNER

SNACKS

Exercise Type:

....

Exercise (Minutes):

Net Carbs: ...... g Proteins: ...... g Fats: ...... g

Net Carbs: ...... g Proteins: ...... g Fats: ...... g

....

DAILY MACROS Net Carbs: ...... g Proteins: ...... g Fats: ...... g

Notes:

DAY 96 | Date: .... Mood Check: 😃 🙂 😐 🙁 ☹️

BREAKFAST

LUNCH

Water:

🥤🥤🥤🥤
🥤🥤🥤🥤

Net Carbs: ...... g Proteins: ...... g Fats: ...... g

Net Carbs: ...... g Proteins: ...... g Fats: ...... g

Sleep (Hours):

....

DINNER

SNACKS

Exercise Type:

....

Exercise (Minutes):

Net Carbs: ...... g Proteins: ...... g Fats: ...... g

Net Carbs: ...... g Proteins: ...... g Fats: ...... g

....

DAILY MACROS Net Carbs: ...... g Proteins: ...... g Fats: ...... g

Notes:

DAY 97 Date: .... Mood Check: 😀 😊 😐 🙁 😟

BREAKFAST	LUNCH	Water:
		🥛🥛🥛🥛🥛 🥛🥛🥛🥛🥛
		Sleep (Hours):
Net Carbs: ...... g Proteins: ...... g Fats: ...... g	Net Carbs: ...... g Proteins: ...... g Fats: ...... g	....
DINNER	SNACKS	Exercise Type:
		....
		Exercise (Minutes):
Net Carbs: ...... g Proteins: ...... g Fats: ...... g	Net Carbs: ...... g Proteins: ...... g Fats: ...... g	....
DAILY MACROS Net Carbs: .... g Proteins: .... g Fats: .... g		

Notes:

DAY 98 Date: .... Mood Check: 😀 😊 😐 🙁 😟

BREAKFAST	LUNCH	Water:
		🥛🥛🥛🥛🥛 🥛🥛🥛🥛🥛
		Sleep (Hours):
Net Carbs: ...... g Proteins: ...... g Fats: ...... g	Net Carbs: ...... g Proteins: ...... g Fats: ...... g	....
DINNER	SNACKS	Exercise Type:
		....
		Exercise (Minutes):
Net Carbs: ...... g Proteins: ...... g Fats: ...... g	Net Carbs: ...... g Proteins: ...... g Fats: ...... g	....
DAILY MACROS Net Carbs: .... g Proteins: .... g Fats: .... g		

Notes:

WEEKLY INTENTIONS

What are you excited for this week?

....

....

....

....

What is something you'd like to work on this week? ....

....

....

....

TARGET MACROS

Carbs: .... %
Proteins: .... %
Fats: .... %

DAY 99 Date: .... Mood Check: ☺ ☺ ☺ ☹ ☹

BREAKFAST	LUNCH	Water:
		🥤🥤🥤🥤🥤 🥤🥤🥤🥤🥤
		Sleep (Hours):
Net Carbs: ...... g Proteins: ...... g Fats: ...... g	Net Carbs: ...... g Proteins: ...... g Fats: ...... g	....
DINNER	SNACKS	Exercise Type: ....
		Exercise (Minutes):
Net Carbs: ...... g Proteins: ...... g Fats: ...... g	Net Carbs: ...... g Proteins: ...... g Fats: ...... g	....

DAILY MACROS   Net Carbs: ...... g   Proteins: ...... g   Fats: ...... g

Notes:

DAY 100   Date: ....   Mood Check: 😃 🙂 😐 🙁 😣

BREAKFAST	LUNCH	Water:
		🥤🥤🥤🥤🥤 🥤🥤🥤🥤🥤
		Sleep (Hours):
Net Carbs: ...... g Proteins: ...... g Fats: ...... g	Net Carbs: ...... g Proteins: ...... g Fats: ...... g	....
DINNER	SNACKS	Exercise Type:
		....
		Exercise (Minutes):
Net Carbs: ...... g Proteins: ...... g Fats: ...... g	Net Carbs: ...... g Proteins: ...... g Fats: ...... g	....
DAILY MACROS Net Carbs: ...... g Proteins: ...... g Fats: ...... g		

Notes:

DAY 101   Date: ....   Mood Check: 😃 🙂 😐 🙁 😣

BREAKFAST	LUNCH	Water:
		🥤🥤🥤🥤🥤 🥤🥤🥤🥤🥤
		Sleep (Hours):
Net Carbs: ...... g Proteins: ...... g Fats: ...... g	Net Carbs: ...... g Proteins: ...... g Fats: ...... g	....
DINNER	SNACKS	Exercise Type:
		....
		Exercise (Minutes):
Net Carbs: ...... g Proteins: ...... g Fats: ...... g	Net Carbs: ...... g Proteins: ...... g Fats: ...... g	....
DAILY MACROS Net Carbs: ...... g Proteins: ...... g Fats: ...... g		

Notes:

DAY 102

Date: .... Mood Check: 😃 🙂 😐 🙁 😫

BREAKFAST

LUNCH

Water:

Sleep (Hours):

Net Carbs: ...... g Proteins: ...... g Fats: ...... g   Net Carbs: ...... g Proteins: ...... g Fats: ...... g   ....

DINNER

SNACKS

Exercise Type:

....

Exercise (Minutes):

Net Carbs: ...... g Proteins: ...... g Fats: ...... g   Net Carbs: ...... g Proteins: ...... g Fats: ...... g

DAILY MACROS   Net Carbs: ...... g   Proteins: ...... g   Fats: ...... g

....

Notes:

DAY 103

Date: .... Mood Check: 😃 🙂 😐 🙁 😫

BREAKFAST

LUNCH

Water:

Sleep (Hours):

Net Carbs: ...... g Proteins: ...... g Fats: ...... g   Net Carbs: ...... g Proteins: ...... g Fats: ...... g   ....

DINNER

SNACKS

Exercise Type:

....

Exercise (Minutes):

Net Carbs: ...... g Proteins: ...... g Fats: ...... g   Net Carbs: ...... g Proteins: ...... g Fats: ...... g

DAILY MACROS   Net Carbs: ...... g   Proteins: ...... g   Fats: ...... g

....

Notes:

DAY 104 Date: .... Mood Check: 😀 🙂 😐 🙁 😣

BREAKFAST	LUNCH	Water: 🥛🥛🥛🥛🥛 🥛🥛🥛🥛🥛
		Sleep (Hours):
Net Carbs: ...... g Proteins: ...... g Fats: ...... g	Net Carbs: ...... g Proteins: ...... g Fats: ...... g	....
DINNER	SNACKS	Exercise Type: .... Exercise (Minutes):
Net Carbs: ...... g Proteins: ...... g Fats: ...... g	Net Carbs: ...... g Proteins: ...... g Fats: ...... g	
DAILY MACROS Net Carbs: ...... g Proteins: ...... g Fats: ...... g		....

Notes:

DAY 105 Date: .... Mood Check: 😀 🙂 😐 🙁 😣

BREAKFAST	LUNCH	Water: 🥛🥛🥛🥛🥛 🥛🥛🥛🥛🥛
		Sleep (Hours):
Net Carbs: ...... g Proteins: ...... g Fats: ...... g	Net Carbs: ...... g Proteins: ...... g Fats: ...... g	....
DINNER	SNACKS	Exercise Type: .... Exercise (Minutes):
Net Carbs: ...... g Proteins: ...... g Fats: ...... g	Net Carbs: ...... g Proteins: ...... g Fats: ...... g	
DAILY MACROS Net Carbs: ...... g Proteins: ...... g Fats: ...... g		....

Notes:

WEEKLY INTENTIONS

What are you excited for this week?

....

....

....

....

What is something you'd like to work on this week? ....

....

....

....

DAY 106	Date:	Mood Check: ☺ ☺ ☺ ☹ ☹

BREAKFAST	LUNCH	Water:
		🥛🥛🥛🥛🥛 🥛🥛🥛🥛🥛
		Sleep (Hours):
Net Carbs: ...... g Proteins: ...... g Fats: ...... g	Net Carbs: ...... g Proteins: ...... g Fats: ...... g	....
DINNER	SNACKS	Exercise Type:
		....
		Exercise (Minutes):
Net Carbs: ...... g Proteins: ...... g Fats: ...... g	Net Carbs: ...... g Proteins: ...... g Fats: ...... g	....
DAILY MACROS	Net Carbs: ...... g Proteins: ...... g Fats: ...... g	

Notes:

DAY 107 Date: .... Mood Check: 😃 😊 😐 😟 😣

BREAKFAST	LUNCH	Water:
		🥤🥤🥤🥤🥤 🥤🥤🥤🥤🥤
		Sleep (Hours):
Net Carbs: ...... g Proteins: ...... g Fats: ...... g	Net Carbs: ...... g Proteins: ...... g Fats: ...... g	....
DINNER	SNACKS	Exercise Type:
		....
		Exercise (Minutes):
Net Carbs: ...... g Proteins: ...... g Fats: ...... g	Net Carbs: ...... g Proteins: ...... g Fats: ...... g	....
DAILY MACROS Net Carbs: ...... g Proteins: ...... g Fats: ...... g		

Notes:

DAY 108 Date: .... Mood Check: 😃 😊 😐 😟 😣

BREAKFAST	LUNCH	Water:
		🥤🥤🥤🥤🥤 🥤🥤🥤🥤🥤
		Sleep (Hours):
Net Carbs: ...... g Proteins: ...... g Fats: ...... g	Net Carbs: ...... g Proteins: ...... g Fats: ...... g	....
DINNER	SNACKS	Exercise Type:
		....
		Exercise (Minutes):
Net Carbs: ...... g Proteins: ...... g Fats: ...... g	Net Carbs: ...... g Proteins: ...... g Fats: ...... g	....
DAILY MACROS Net Carbs: ...... g Proteins: ...... g Fats: ...... g		

Notes:

DAY 109   Date: ....   Mood Check: 😃 😊 😐 😕 😞

BREAKFAST

LUNCH

Water:

🥤🥤🥤🥤🥤
🥤🥤🥤🥤🥤

Sleep (Hours):

Net Carbs: ...... g Proteins: ...... g Fats: ...... g | Net Carbs: ...... g Proteins: ...... g Fats: ...... g

....

DINNER

SNACKS

Exercise
Type:

....

Exercise
(Minutes):

Net Carbs: ...... g Proteins: ...... g Fats: ...... g | Net Carbs: ...... g Proteins: ...... g Fats: ...... g

....

DAILY MACROS   Net Carbs: .... g   Proteins: .... g   Fats: .... g

Notes:

DAY 110   Date: ....   Mood Check: 😃 😊 😐 😕 😞

BREAKFAST

LUNCH

Water:

🥤🥤🥤🥤🥤
🥤🥤🥤🥤🥤

Sleep (Hours):

Net Carbs: ...... g Proteins: ...... g Fats: ...... g | Net Carbs: ...... g Proteins: ...... g Fats: ...... g

....

DINNER

SNACKS

Exercise
Type:

....

Exercise
(Minutes):

Net Carbs: ...... g Proteins: ...... g Fats: ...... g | Net Carbs: ...... g Proteins: ...... g Fats: ...... g

....

DAILY MACROS   Net Carbs: .... g   Proteins: .... g   Fats: .... g

Notes:

DAY 111

Date: .... Mood Check: 😃 🙂 😐 🙁 😣

BREAKFAST	LUNCH	Water:
		🥛🥛🥛🥛🥛 🥛🥛🥛🥛🥛
		Sleep (Hours):
Net Carbs: ...... g Proteins: ...... g Fats: ...... g	Net Carbs: ...... g Proteins: ...... g Fats: ...... g	....

DINNER	SNACKS	Exercise Type:
		....
		Exercise (Minutes):
Net Carbs: ...... g Proteins: ...... g Fats: ...... g	Net Carbs: ...... g Proteins: ...... g Fats: ...... g	
DAILY MACROS Net Carbs: ...... g Proteins: ...... g Fats: ...... g		....

Notes:

DAY 112

Date: .... Mood Check: 😃 🙂 😐 🙁 😣

BREAKFAST	LUNCH	Water:
		🥛🥛🥛🥛🥛 🥛🥛🥛🥛🥛
		Sleep (Hours):
Net Carbs: ...... g Proteins: ...... g Fats: ...... g	Net Carbs: ...... g Proteins: ...... g Fats: ...... g	....

DINNER	SNACKS	Exercise Type:
		....
		Exercise (Minutes):
Net Carbs: ...... g Proteins: ...... g Fats: ...... g	Net Carbs: ...... g Proteins: ...... g Fats: ...... g	
DAILY MACROS Net Carbs: ...... g Proteins: ...... g Fats: ...... g		....

Notes:

MEASUREMENT	CURRENT	MONTH CHANGE
WEIGHT (LBS)		
UPPER ARMS (IN)		
CHEST (IN)		
WAIST (IN)		
HIPS (IN)		
THIGHS (IN)		
CALVES (IN)		

CHECKING IN

Congratulations on making it this far! What are you most proud of from the past 4 weeks?

....

....

....

....

....

What was your biggest challenge over the past 4 weeks?

....

....

....

....

....

What are some goals you would like to work toward over the
next 4 weeks?

....

....

....

....

....

Reflect on your mood over the past month—did you notice
differences related to your eating habits?

....

....

....

....

....

WEEKLY INTENTIONS

What are you excited for this week?

....

....

....

Carbs: .... %
Proteins: .... %
Fats: .... %

What is something you'd like to work on this week? ....

....

....

....

DAY 113	Date:	Mood Check: 😃 🙂 😐 🙁 ☹️

BREAKFAST

LUNCH

Water:

🥛🥛🥛🥛
🥛🥛🥛🥛

Net Carbs: ...... g Proteins: ...... g Fats: ...... g

Net Carbs: ...... g Proteins: ...... g Fats: ...... g

Sleep (Hours):

....

DINNER

SNACKS

Exercise Type:

....

Exercise (Minutes):

Net Carbs: ...... g Proteins: ...... g Fats: ...... g

Net Carbs: ...... g Proteins: ...... g Fats: ...... g

....

DAILY MACROS   Net Carbs: ...... g   Proteins: ...... g   Fats: ...... g

Notes:

DAY 114 Date: .... Mood Check: 😃 ☺ 😐 🙁 ☹

BREAKFAST	LUNCH	Water:
		🥤🥤🥤🥤🥤 🥤🥤🥤🥤🥤
		Sleep (Hours):
Net Carbs: ...... g Proteins: ...... g Fats: ...... g	Net Carbs: ...... g Proteins: ...... g Fats: ...... g	....
DINNER	**SNACKS**	Exercise Type:
		....
		Exercise (Minutes):
Net Carbs: ...... g Proteins: ...... g Fats: ...... g	Net Carbs: ...... g Proteins: ...... g Fats: ...... g	....
DAILY MACROS Net Carbs: ...... g Proteins: ...... g Fats: ...... g		

Notes:

DAY 115 Date: .... Mood Check: 😃 ☺ 😐 🙁 ☹

BREAKFAST	LUNCH	Water:
		🥤🥤🥤🥤🥤 🥤🥤🥤🥤🥤
		Sleep (Hours):
Net Carbs: ...... g Proteins: ...... g Fats: ...... g	Net Carbs: ...... g Proteins: ...... g Fats: ...... g	....
DINNER	**SNACKS**	Exercise Type:
		....
		Exercise (Minutes):
Net Carbs: ...... g Proteins: ...... g Fats: ...... g	Net Carbs: ...... g Proteins: ...... g Fats: ...... g	....
DAILY MACROS Net Carbs: ...... g Proteins: ...... g Fats: ...... g		

Notes:

DAY 116 | Date: .... Mood Check: 😄 🙂 😐 🙁 😟

BREAKFAST

LUNCH

Water:

Net Carbs: ...... g Proteins: ...... g Fats: ...... g | Net Carbs: ...... g Proteins: ...... g Fats: ...... g

Sleep (Hours):

....

DINNER

SNACKS

Exercise Type:

....

Exercise (Minutes):

Net Carbs: ...... g Proteins: ...... g Fats: ...... g | Net Carbs: ...... g Proteins: ...... g Fats: ...... g

....

DAILY MACROS Net Carbs: ...... g Proteins: ...... g Fats: ...... g

Notes:

DAY 117 | Date: .... Mood Check: 😄 🙂 😐 🙁 😟

BREAKFAST

LUNCH

Water:

Net Carbs: ...... g Proteins: ...... g Fats: ...... g | Net Carbs: ...... g Proteins: ...... g Fats: ...... g

Sleep (Hours):

....

DINNER

SNACKS

Exercise Type:

....

Exercise (Minutes):

Net Carbs: ...... g Proteins: ...... g Fats: ...... g | Net Carbs: ...... g Proteins: ...... g Fats: ...... g

....

DAILY MACROS Net Carbs: ...... g Proteins: ...... g Fats: ...... g

Notes:

DAY 118

Date: .... Mood Check: ☺ ☺ 😐 ☹ 😞

BREAKFAST	LUNCH	Water:
		🥤🥤🥤🥤🥤 🥤🥤🥤🥤🥤
		Sleep (Hours):
Net Carbs: ...... g Proteins: ...... g Fats: ...... g	Net Carbs: ...... g Proteins: ...... g Fats: ...... g	....
DINNER	**SNACKS**	Exercise Type:
		....
		Exercise (Minutes):
Net Carbs: ...... g Proteins: ...... g Fats: ...... g	Net Carbs: ...... g Proteins: ...... g Fats: ...... g	....
DAILY MACROS Net Carbs: ...... g Proteins: ...... g Fats: ...... g		

Notes:

DAY 119

Date: .... Mood Check: ☺ ☺ 😐 ☹ 😞

BREAKFAST	LUNCH	Water:
		🥤🥤🥤🥤🥤 🥤🥤🥤🥤🥤
		Sleep (Hours):
Net Carbs: ...... g Proteins: ...... g Fats: ...... g	Net Carbs: ...... g Proteins: ...... g Fats: ...... g	....
DINNER	**SNACKS**	Exercise Type:
		....
		Exercise (Minutes):
Net Carbs: ...... g Proteins: ...... g Fats: ...... g	Net Carbs: ...... g Proteins: ...... g Fats: ...... g	....
DAILY MACROS Net Carbs: ...... g Proteins: ...... g Fats: ...... g		

Notes:

WEEKLY INTENTIONS

What are you excited for this week?

Carbs: .... %
Proteins: .... %
Fats: .... %

....

....

....

What is something you'd like to work on this week? ....

....

....

....

DAY 120	Date:	Mood Check: 😃 🙂 😐 🙁 ☹️
BREAKFAST	**LUNCH**	Water:
Net Carbs: ...... g Proteins: ...... g Fats: ...... g	Net Carbs: ...... g Proteins: ...... g Fats: ...... g	Sleep (Hours): ....
DINNER	**SNACKS**	Exercise Type: .... Exercise (Minutes):
Net Carbs: ...... g Proteins: ...... g Fats: ...... g	Net Carbs: ...... g Proteins: ...... g Fats: ...... g	....
DAILY MACROS	Net Carbs: ...... g Proteins: ...... g Fats: ...... g	

Notes:

DAY 121	Date:..	Mood Check: 😄 🙂 😐 🙁 😣	
BREAKFAST	**LUNCH**	**Water:**
		🥤🥤🥤🥤🥤 🥤🥤🥤🥤🥤
		Sleep (Hours):
Net Carbs: ...... g Proteins: ...... g Fats: ...... g	Net Carbs: ...... g Proteins: ...... g Fats: ...... g	....
DINNER	**SNACKS**	**Exercise Type:**
		....
		Exercise (Minutes):
Net Carbs: ...... g Proteins: ...... g Fats: ...... g	Net Carbs: ...... g Proteins: ...... g Fats: ...... g	
DAILY MACROS Net Carbs: .... g Proteins: .... g Fats: .... g		....

Notes:

DAY 122	Date:..	Mood Check: 😄 🙂 😐 🙁 😣	
BREAKFAST	**LUNCH**	**Water:**
		🥤🥤🥤🥤🥤 🥤🥤🥤🥤🥤
		Sleep (Hours):
Net Carbs: ...... g Proteins: ...... g Fats: ...... g	Net Carbs: ...... g Proteins: ...... g Fats: ...... g	....
DINNER	**SNACKS**	**Exercise Type:**
		....
		Exercise (Minutes):
Net Carbs: ...... g Proteins: ...... g Fats: ...... g	Net Carbs: ...... g Proteins: ...... g Fats: ...... g	
DAILY MACROS Net Carbs: .... g Proteins: .... g Fats: .... g		....

Notes:

DAY 123   Date: ....   Mood Check: 😀 😊 😐 🙁 😣

BREAKFAST	LUNCH	Water:
		🥛🥛🥛🥛🥛 🥛🥛🥛🥛🥛
		Sleep (Hours):
Net Carbs: ...... g Proteins: ...... g Fats: ...... g	Net Carbs: ...... g Proteins: ...... g Fats: ...... g	....
DINNER	SNACKS	Exercise Type:
		....
		Exercise (Minutes):
Net Carbs: ...... g Proteins: ...... g Fats: ...... g	Net Carbs: ...... g Proteins: ...... g Fats: ...... g	....
DAILY MACROS Net Carbs: .... g Proteins: .... g Fats: .... g		

Notes:

DAY 124   Date: ....   Mood Check: 😀 😊 😐 🙁 😣

BREAKFAST	LUNCH	Water:
		🥛🥛🥛🥛🥛 🥛🥛🥛🥛🥛
		Sleep (Hours):
Net Carbs: ...... g Proteins: ...... g Fats: ...... g	Net Carbs: ...... g Proteins: ...... g Fats: ...... g	....
DINNER	SNACKS	Exercise Type:
		....
		Exercise (Minutes):
Net Carbs: ...... g Proteins: ...... g Fats: ...... g	Net Carbs: ...... g Proteins: ...... g Fats: ...... g	....
DAILY MACROS Net Carbs: .... g Proteins: .... g Fats: .... g		

Notes:

DAY 125   Date: ....   Mood Check: 😀 😊 😐 🙁 ☹️

BREAKFAST	LUNCH	Water:
		🥤🥤🥤🥤🥤 🥤🥤🥤🥤🥤
		Sleep (Hours):
Net Carbs: ...... g Proteins: ...... g Fats: ...... g	Net Carbs: ...... g Proteins: ...... g Fats: ...... g	....
DINNER	SNACKS	Exercise Type:
		....
		Exercise (Minutes):
Net Carbs: ...... g Proteins: ...... g Fats: ...... g	Net Carbs: ...... g Proteins: ...... g Fats: ...... g	....

DAILY MACROS   Net Carbs: ...... g   Proteins: ...... g   Fats: ...... g

Notes:

DAY 126   Date: ....   Mood Check: 😀 😊 😐 🙁 ☹️

BREAKFAST	LUNCH	Water:
		🥤🥤🥤🥤🥤 🥤🥤🥤🥤🥤
		Sleep (Hours):
Net Carbs: ...... g Proteins: ...... g Fats: ...... g	Net Carbs: ...... g Proteins: ...... g Fats: ...... g	....
DINNER	SNACKS	Exercise Type:
		....
		Exercise (Minutes):
Net Carbs: ...... g Proteins: ...... g Fats: ...... g	Net Carbs: ...... g Proteins: ...... g Fats: ...... g	....

DAILY MACROS   Net Carbs: ...... g   Proteins: ...... g   Fats: ...... g

Notes:

WEEKLY INTENTIONS

What are you excited for this week?

Carbs: .... %
Proteins: .... %
Fats: .... %

....

....

....

....

What is something you'd like to work on this week? ....

....

....

....

DAY 127 Date: .... Mood Check: 😀 🙂 😐 🙁 😟

BREAKFAST	LUNCH	Water:
		🥤🥤🥤🥤🥤 🥤🥤🥤🥤🥤
		Sleep (Hours):
Net Carbs: ...... g Proteins: ...... g Fats: ...... g	Net Carbs: ...... g Proteins: ...... g Fats: ...... g	....
DINNER	SNACKS	Exercise Type: ....
		Exercise (Minutes):
Net Carbs: ...... g Proteins: ...... g Fats: ...... g	Net Carbs: ...... g Proteins: ...... g Fats: ...... g	
DAILY MACROS Net Carbs: ...... g Proteins: ...... g Fats: ...... g		....

Notes:

DAY 128 Date: .... Mood Check: 😀 😊 😐 🙁 ☹️

BREAKFAST	LUNCH	Water:
		🥛🥛🥛🥛 🥛🥛🥛🥛
		Sleep (Hours):
Net Carbs: ...... g Proteins: ...... g Fats: ...... g	Net Carbs: ...... g Proteins: ...... g Fats: ...... g	....
DINNER	**SNACKS**	Exercise Type:
		....
		Exercise (Minutes):
Net Carbs: ...... g Proteins: ...... g Fats: ...... g	Net Carbs: ...... g Proteins: ...... g Fats: ...... g	....
DAILY MACROS Net Carbs: ...... g Proteins: ...... g Fats: ...... g		

Notes:

DAY 129 Date: .... Mood Check: 😀 😊 😐 🙁 ☹️

BREAKFAST	LUNCH	Water:
		🥛🥛🥛🥛 🥛🥛🥛🥛
		Sleep (Hours):
Net Carbs: ...... g Proteins: ...... g Fats: ...... g	Net Carbs: ...... g Proteins: ...... g Fats: ...... g	....
DINNER	**SNACKS**	Exercise Type:
		....
		Exercise (Minutes):
Net Carbs: ...... g Proteins: ...... g Fats: ...... g	Net Carbs: ...... g Proteins: ...... g Fats: ...... g	....
DAILY MACROS Net Carbs: ...... g Proteins: ...... g Fats: ...... g		

Notes:

DAY 130

Date: .... Mood Check: 😃 😊 😐 🙁 ☹️

BREAKFAST

LUNCH

Water:

Sleep (Hours):

Net Carbs: ...... g Proteins: ...... g Fats: ...... g   Net Carbs: ...... g Proteins: ...... g Fats: ...... g   ....

DINNER

SNACKS

Exercise Type:

....

Exercise (Minutes):

Net Carbs: ...... g Proteins: ...... g Fats: ...... g   Net Carbs: ...... g Proteins: ...... g Fats: ...... g   ....

DAILY MACROS   Net Carbs: ...... g   Proteins: ...... g   Fats: ...... g

Notes:

DAY 131

Date: .... Mood Check: 😃 😊 😐 🙁 ☹️

BREAKFAST

LUNCH

Water:

Sleep (Hours):

Net Carbs: ...... g Proteins: ...... g Fats: ...... g   Net Carbs: ...... g Proteins: ...... g Fats: ...... g   ....

DINNER

SNACKS

Exercise Type:

....

Exercise (Minutes):

Net Carbs: ...... g Proteins: ...... g Fats: ...... g   Net Carbs: ...... g Proteins: ...... g Fats: ...... g   ....

DAILY MACROS   Net Carbs: ...... g   Proteins: ...... g   Fats: ...... g

Notes:

DAY 132 Date: .... Mood Check: 😀 🙂 😐 🙁 😞

BREAKFAST	LUNCH	Water:
		🥛🥛🥛🥛🥛 🥛🥛🥛🥛🥛
		Sleep (Hours):
Net Carbs: ...... g Proteins: ...... g Fats: ...... g	Net Carbs: ...... g Proteins: ...... g Fats: ...... g	....
DINNER	**SNACKS**	Exercise Type:
		....
		Exercise (Minutes):
Net Carbs: ...... g Proteins: ...... g Fats: ...... g	Net Carbs: ...... g Proteins: ...... g Fats: ...... g	....
DAILY MACROS Net Carbs: ...... g Proteins: ...... g Fats: ...... g		

Notes:

DAY 133 Date: .... Mood Check: 😀 🙂 😐 🙁 😞

BREAKFAST	LUNCH	Water:
		🥛🥛🥛🥛🥛 🥛🥛🥛🥛🥛
		Sleep (Hours):
Net Carbs: ...... g Proteins: ...... g Fats: ...... g	Net Carbs: ...... g Proteins: ...... g Fats: ...... g	....
DINNER	**SNACKS**	Exercise Type:
		....
		Exercise (Minutes):
Net Carbs: ...... g Proteins: ...... g Fats: ...... g	Net Carbs: ...... g Proteins: ...... g Fats: ...... g	....
DAILY MACROS Net Carbs: ...... g Proteins: ...... g Fats: ...... g		

Notes:

WEEKLY INTENTIONS

What are you excited for this week?

....

....

....

....

Carbs: .... %
Proteins: .... %
Fats: .... %

What is something you'd like to work on this week? ....

....

....

....

DAY 134	Date:	Mood Check: ☺ ☺ 😐 🙁 ☹

BREAKFAST	LUNCH	Water:
		🥛🥛🥛🥛🥛 🥛🥛🥛🥛🥛
		Sleep (Hours):
Net Carbs: ...... g Proteins: ...... g Fats: ...... g	Net Carbs: ...... g Proteins: ...... g Fats: ...... g	....
DINNER	SNACKS	Exercise Type: .... Exercise (Minutes):
Net Carbs: ...... g Proteins: ...... g Fats: ...... g	Net Carbs: ...... g Proteins: ...... g Fats: ...... g	....
DAILY MACROS	Net Carbs: ...... g Proteins: ...... g Fats: ...... g	

Notes:

DAY 135 | Date: .... Mood Check: 😀 🙂 😐 🙁 ☹️

BREAKFAST	LUNCH	Water:
		🥛🥛🥛🥛🥛 🥛🥛🥛🥛🥛
		Sleep (Hours):
Net Carbs: ...... g Proteins: ...... g Fats: ...... g	Net Carbs: ...... g Proteins: ...... g Fats: ...... g	....
DINNER	**SNACKS**	Exercise Type:
		....
		Exercise (Minutes):
Net Carbs: ...... g Proteins: ...... g Fats: ...... g	Net Carbs: ...... g Proteins: ...... g Fats: ...... g	....
DAILY MACROS Net Carbs: ...... g Proteins: ...... g Fats: ...... g		

Notes:

DAY 136 | Date: .... Mood Check: 😀 🙂 😐 🙁 ☹️

BREAKFAST	LUNCH	Water:
		🥛🥛🥛🥛🥛 🥛🥛🥛🥛🥛
		Sleep (Hours):
Net Carbs: ...... g Proteins: ...... g Fats: ...... g	Net Carbs: ...... g Proteins: ...... g Fats: ...... g	....
DINNER	**SNACKS**	Exercise Type:
		....
		Exercise (Minutes):
Net Carbs: ...... g Proteins: ...... g Fats: ...... g	Net Carbs: ...... g Proteins: ...... g Fats: ...... g	....
DAILY MACROS Net Carbs: ...... g Proteins: ...... g Fats: ...... g		

Notes:

DAY 137 Date: .... Mood Check: 😀 😊 😐 🙁 ☹️

BREAKFAST

Net Carbs: ...... g Proteins: ...... g Fats: ...... g

DINNER

Net Carbs: ...... g Proteins: ...... g Fats: ...... g

LUNCH

Net Carbs: ...... g Proteins: ...... g Fats: ...... g

SNACKS

Net Carbs: ...... g Proteins: ...... g Fats: ...... g

Water:

Sleep (Hours):

....

Exercise Type:

....

Exercise (Minutes):

....

DAILY MACROS Net Carbs: ...... g Proteins: ...... g Fats: ...... g

Notes:

DAY 138 Date: .... Mood Check: 😀 😊 😐 🙁 ☹️

BREAKFAST

Net Carbs: ...... g Proteins: ...... g Fats: ...... g

DINNER

Net Carbs: ...... g Proteins: ...... g Fats: ...... g

LUNCH

Net Carbs: ...... g Proteins: ...... g Fats: ...... g

SNACKS

Net Carbs: ...... g Proteins: ...... g Fats: ...... g

Water:

Sleep (Hours):

....

Exercise Type:

....

Exercise (Minutes):

....

DAILY MACROS Net Carbs: ...... g Proteins: ...... g Fats: ...... g

Notes:

DAY 139

Date: ....   Mood Check: 😀 🙂 😐 🙁 ☹️

BREAKFAST	LUNCH	Water:
		🥤🥤🥤🥤🥤
		🥤🥤🥤🥤🥤
		Sleep (Hours):
Net Carbs: ...... g Proteins: ...... g Fats: ...... g	Net Carbs: ...... g Proteins: ...... g Fats: ...... g	....

DINNER	SNACKS	Exercise Type:
		....
		Exercise (Minutes):
Net Carbs: ...... g Proteins: ...... g Fats: ...... g	Net Carbs: ...... g Proteins: ...... g Fats: ...... g	

DAILY MACROS   Net Carbs: .... g   Proteins: .... g   Fats: .... g

Notes:

DAY 140

Date: ....   Mood Check: 😀 🙂 😐 🙁 ☹️

BREAKFAST	LUNCH	Water:
		🥤🥤🥤🥤🥤
		🥤🥤🥤🥤🥤
		Sleep (Hours):
Net Carbs: ...... g Proteins: ...... g Fats: ...... g	Net Carbs: ...... g Proteins: ...... g Fats: ...... g	....

DINNER	SNACKS	Exercise Type:
		....
		Exercise (Minutes):
Net Carbs: ...... g Proteins: ...... g Fats: ...... g	Net Carbs: ...... g Proteins: ...... g Fats: ...... g	

DAILY MACROS   Net Carbs: .... g   Proteins: .... g   Fats: .... g

Notes:

MEASUREMENT	CURRENT	MONTH CHANGE
WEIGHT (LBS)		
UPPER ARMS (IN)		
CHEST (IN)		
WAIST (IN)		
HIPS (IN)		
THIGHS (IN)		
CALVES (IN)		

CHECKING IN

Congratulations on making it this far! What are you most proud of from the past 4 weeks?

....

....

....

....

....

What was your biggest challenge over the past 4 weeks?

....

....

....

....

....

....

What are some goals you would like to work toward over the next 4 weeks?

....

....

....

....

....

....

Reflect on your mood over the past month—did you notice differences related to your eating habits?

....

....

....

....

....

WEEKLY INTENTIONS

What are you excited for this week?

....

....

....

....

What is something you'd like to work on this week? ....

....

....

....

DAY 141	Date:	Mood Check: 😃 🙂 😐 🙁 😞

BREAKFAST	LUNCH	Water:
		🥛🥛🥛🥛 🥛🥛🥛🥛
		Sleep (Hours):
Net Carbs: ...... g Proteins: ...... g Fats: ...... g	Net Carbs: ...... g Proteins: ...... g Fats: ...... g	....
DINNER	SNACKS	Exercise Type:
		....
		Exercise (Minutes):
Net Carbs: ...... g Proteins: ...... g Fats: ...... g	Net Carbs: ...... g Proteins: ...... g Fats: ...... g	....
DAILY MACROS	Net Carbs: ...... g Proteins: ...... g Fats: ...... g	

Notes:

DAY 142 Date: .... Mood Check: 😃 😊 😐 🙁 😖

BREAKFAST	LUNCH	Water:
		🥛🥛🥛🥛🥛 🥛🥛🥛🥛🥛
		Sleep (Hours):
Net Carbs: ...... g Proteins: ...... g Fats: ...... g	Net Carbs: ...... g Proteins: ...... g Fats: ...... g	....
DINNER	SNACKS	Exercise Type:
		....
		Exercise (Minutes):
Net Carbs: ...... g Proteins: ...... g Fats: ...... g	Net Carbs: ...... g Proteins: ...... g Fats: ...... g	....
DAILY MACROS Net Carbs: ...... g Proteins: ...... g Fats: ...... g		

Notes:

DAY 143 Date: .... Mood Check: 😃 😊 😐 🙁 😖

BREAKFAST	LUNCH	Water:
		🥛🥛🥛🥛🥛 🥛🥛🥛🥛🥛
		Sleep (Hours):
Net Carbs: ...... g Proteins: ...... g Fats: ...... g	Net Carbs: ...... g Proteins: ...... g Fats: ...... g	....
DINNER	SNACKS	Exercise Type:
		....
		Exercise (Minutes):
Net Carbs: ...... g Proteins: ...... g Fats: ...... g	Net Carbs: ...... g Proteins: ...... g Fats: ...... g	....
DAILY MACROS Net Carbs: ...... g Proteins: ...... g Fats: ...... g		

Notes:

DAY 144 Date: .... Mood Check: 😀 😊 😐 🙁 😞

BREAKFAST

LUNCH

Water:

Sleep (Hours):

Net Carbs: ...... g Proteins: ...... g Fats: ...... g | Net Carbs: ...... g Proteins: ...... g Fats: ...... g | ....

DINNER

SNACKS

Exercise Type:

....

Exercise (Minutes):

Net Carbs: ...... g Proteins: ...... g Fats: ...... g | Net Carbs: ...... g Proteins: ...... g Fats: ...... g | ....

DAILY MACROS Net Carbs: ...... g Proteins: ...... g Fats: ...... g

Notes:

DAY 145 Date: .... Mood Check: 😀 😊 😐 🙁 😞

BREAKFAST

LUNCH

Water:

Sleep (Hours):

Net Carbs: ...... g Proteins: ...... g Fats: ...... g | Net Carbs: ...... g Proteins: ...... g Fats: ...... g | ....

DINNER

SNACKS

Exercise Type:

....

Exercise (Minutes):

Net Carbs: ...... g Proteins: ...... g Fats: ...... g | Net Carbs: ...... g Proteins: ...... g Fats: ...... g | ....

DAILY MACROS Net Carbs: ...... g Proteins: ...... g Fats: ...... g

Notes:

DAY 146　Date: .... Mood Check: 😃 😊 😐 🙁 😣

BREAKFAST	LUNCH	Water:
		🥤🥤🥤🥤 🥤🥤🥤🥤
		Sleep (Hours):
Net Carbs: ...... g Proteins: ...... g Fats: ...... g	Net Carbs: ...... g Proteins: ...... g Fats: ...... g	....
DINNER	**SNACKS**	Exercise Type:
		....
		Exercise (Minutes):
Net Carbs: ...... g Proteins: ...... g Fats: ...... g	Net Carbs: ...... g Proteins: ...... g Fats: ...... g	....
DAILY MACROS　　Net Carbs: ...... g　　Proteins: ...... g　　Fats: ...... g		

Notes:

DAY 147　Date: .... Mood Check: 😃 😊 😐 🙁 😣

BREAKFAST	LUNCH	Water:
		🥤🥤🥤🥤 🥤🥤🥤🥤
		Sleep (Hours):
Net Carbs: ...... g Proteins: ...... g Fats: ...... g	Net Carbs: ...... g Proteins: ...... g Fats: ...... g	....
DINNER	**SNACKS**	Exercise Type:
		....
		Exercise (Minutes):
Net Carbs: ...... g Proteins: ...... g Fats: ...... g	Net Carbs: ...... g Proteins: ...... g Fats: ...... g	....
DAILY MACROS　　Net Carbs: ...... g　　Proteins: ...... g　　Fats: ...... g		

Notes:

WEEKLY INTENTIONS

What are you excited for this week?

....

....

....

What is something you'd like to work on this week? ....

....

....

....

DAY 148	Date:	Mood Check: 😀 🙂 😐 🙁 ☹️

BREAKFAST	LUNCH	Water:
		🥛🥛🥛🥛🥛 🥛🥛🥛🥛🥛
Net Carbs: ...... g Proteins: ...... g Fats: ...... g	Net Carbs: ...... g Proteins: ...... g Fats: ...... g	Sleep (Hours): ....
DINNER	SNACKS	Exercise Type: .... Exercise (Minutes):
Net Carbs: ...... g Proteins: ...... g Fats: ...... g	Net Carbs: ...... g Proteins: ...... g Fats: ...... g	....
DAILY MACROS	Net Carbs: ...... g Proteins: ...... g Fats: ...... g	

Notes:

DAY 149 Date: .... Mood Check: ☺ ☺ ☺ ☹ ☹

BREAKFAST	LUNCH	Water:
		🥤🥤🥤🥤🥤 🥤🥤🥤🥤🥤
		Sleep (Hours):
Net Carbs: ...... g Proteins: ...... g Fats: ...... g	Net Carbs: ...... g Proteins: ...... g Fats: ...... g	....
DINNER	**SNACKS**	Exercise Type:
		....
		Exercise (Minutes):
Net Carbs: ...... g Proteins: ...... g Fats: ...... g	Net Carbs: ...... g Proteins: ...... g Fats: ...... g	....

DAILY MACROS   Net Carbs: ...... g   Proteins: ...... g   Fats: ...... g

Notes:

DAY 150 Date: .... Mood Check: ☺ ☺ ☺ ☹ ☹

BREAKFAST	LUNCH	Water:
		🥤🥤🥤🥤🥤 🥤🥤🥤🥤🥤
		Sleep (Hours):
Net Carbs: ...... g Proteins: ...... g Fats: ...... g	Net Carbs: ...... g Proteins: ...... g Fats: ...... g	....
DINNER	**SNACKS**	Exercise Type:
		....
		Exercise (Minutes):
Net Carbs: ...... g Proteins: ...... g Fats: ...... g	Net Carbs: ...... g Proteins: ...... g Fats: ...... g	....

DAILY MACROS   Net Carbs: ...... g   Proteins: ...... g   Fats: ...... g

Notes:

DAY 151 Date: .... Mood Check: 😃 😊 😐 😕 ☹️

BREAKFAST

LUNCH

Water:

Net Carbs: ...... g Proteins: ...... g Fats: ...... g   Net Carbs: ...... g Proteins: ...... g Fats: ...... g

Sleep (Hours):

....

DINNER

SNACKS

Exercise Type:

....

Exercise (Minutes):

Net Carbs: ...... g Proteins: ...... g Fats: ...... g   Net Carbs: ...... g Proteins: ...... g Fats: ...... g

....

DAILY MACROS   Net Carbs: ...... g   Proteins: ...... g   Fats: ...... g

Notes:

DAY 152 Date: .... Mood Check: 😃 😊 😐 😕 ☹️

BREAKFAST

LUNCH

Water:

Net Carbs: ...... g Proteins: ...... g Fats: ...... g   Net Carbs: ...... g Proteins: ...... g Fats: ...... g

Sleep (Hours):

....

DINNER

SNACKS

Exercise Type:

....

Exercise (Minutes):

Net Carbs: ...... g Proteins: ...... g Fats: ...... g   Net Carbs: ...... g Proteins: ...... g Fats: ...... g

....

DAILY MACROS   Net Carbs: ...... g   Proteins: ...... g   Fats: ...... g

Notes:

DAY 153 | Date: .... Mood Check: 😊 🙂 😐 🙁 ☹️

BREAKFAST	**LUNCH**	Water:
		🥛🥛🥛🥛 🥛🥛🥛🥛
		Sleep (Hours):
Net Carbs: ...... g Proteins: ...... g Fats: ...... g	Net Carbs: ...... g Proteins: ...... g Fats: ...... g	....
DINNER	**SNACKS**	Exercise Type:
		....
		Exercise (Minutes):
Net Carbs: ...... g Proteins: ...... g Fats: ...... g	Net Carbs: ...... g Proteins: ...... g Fats: ...... g	....
DAILY MACROS Net Carbs: ...... g Proteins: ...... g Fats: ...... g		

Notes:

DAY 154 | Date: .... Mood Check: 😊 🙂 😐 🙁 ☹️

BREAKFAST	**LUNCH**	Water:
		🥛🥛🥛🥛 🥛🥛🥛🥛
		Sleep (Hours):
Net Carbs: ...... g Proteins: ...... g Fats: ...... g	Net Carbs: ...... g Proteins: ...... g Fats: ...... g	....
DINNER	**SNACKS**	Exercise Type:
		....
		Exercise (Minutes):
Net Carbs: ...... g Proteins: ...... g Fats: ...... g	Net Carbs: ...... g Proteins: ...... g Fats: ...... g	....
DAILY MACROS Net Carbs: ...... g Proteins: ...... g Fats: ...... g		

Notes:

WEEKLY INTENTIONS

What are you excited for this week?

....

....

....

....

What is something you'd like to work on this week? ....

....

....

....

DAY 155	Date:	Mood Check: 😃 😊 😐 🙁 ☹️

BREAKFAST	LUNCH	Water:
		🥛🥛🥛🥛🥛
		🥛🥛🥛🥛🥛
		Sleep (Hours):
Net Carbs: ...... g Proteins: ...... g Fats: ...... g	Net Carbs: ...... g Proteins: ...... g Fats: ...... g	....
DINNER	SNACKS	Exercise Type:
		....
		Exercise (Minutes):
Net Carbs: ...... g Proteins: ...... g Fats: ...... g	Net Carbs: ...... g Proteins: ...... g Fats: ...... g	....
DAILY MACROS	Net Carbs: ...... g Proteins: ...... g Fats: ...... g	

Notes:

DAY 156

Date: ....

Mood Check: 😃 🙂 😐 🙁 ☹️

BREAKFAST	LUNCH	Water:
		🥤🥤🥤🥤🥤 🥤🥤🥤🥤🥤
		Sleep (Hours):
Net Carbs: ...... g Proteins: ...... g Fats: ...... g	Net Carbs: ...... g Proteins: ...... g Fats: ...... g	
DINNER	**SNACKS**	Exercise Type: ....
		Exercise (Minutes):
Net Carbs: ...... g Proteins: ...... g Fats: ...... g	Net Carbs: ...... g Proteins: ...... g Fats: ...... g	
DAILY MACROS Net Carbs: ...... g Proteins: ...... g Fats: ...... g		....

Notes:

DAY 157

Date: ....

Mood Check: 😃 🙂 😐 🙁 ☹️

BREAKFAST	LUNCH	Water:
		🥤🥤🥤🥤🥤 🥤🥤🥤🥤🥤
		Sleep (Hours):
Net Carbs: ...... g Proteins: ...... g Fats: ...... g	Net Carbs: ...... g Proteins: ...... g Fats: ...... g	
DINNER	**SNACKS**	Exercise Type: ....
		Exercise (Minutes):
Net Carbs: ...... g Proteins: ...... g Fats: ...... g	Net Carbs: ...... g Proteins: ...... g Fats: ...... g	
DAILY MACROS Net Carbs: ...... g Proteins: ...... g Fats: ...... g		....

Notes:

DAY 158

Date: .... Mood Check: 😀 😊 😐 🙁 ☹️

BREAKFAST

LUNCH

Water:

Net Carbs: ...... g Proteins: ...... g Fats: ...... g

Net Carbs: ...... g Proteins: ...... g Fats: ...... g

Sleep (Hours):

....

DINNER

SNACKS

Exercise Type:

....

Exercise (Minutes):

Net Carbs: ...... g Proteins: ...... g Fats: ...... g

Net Carbs: ...... g Proteins: ...... g Fats: ...... g

....

DAILY MACROS Net Carbs: ...... g Proteins: ...... g Fats: ...... g

Notes:

DAY 159

Date: .... Mood Check: 😀 😊 😐 🙁 ☹️

BREAKFAST

LUNCH

Water:

Net Carbs: ...... g Proteins: ...... g Fats: ...... g

Net Carbs: ...... g Proteins: ...... g Fats: ...... g

Sleep (Hours):

....

DINNER

SNACKS

Exercise Type:

....

Exercise (Minutes):

Net Carbs: ...... g Proteins: ...... g Fats: ...... g

Net Carbs: ...... g Proteins: ...... g Fats: ...... g

....

DAILY MACROS Net Carbs: ...... g Proteins: ...... g Fats: ...... g

Notes:

DAY 160 Date: .... Mood Check: 😀 😊 😐 🙁 ☹️

BREAKFAST	LUNCH	Water:
		🥤🥤🥤🥤🥤 🥤🥤🥤🥤🥤
		Sleep (Hours):
Net Carbs: ...... g Proteins: ...... g Fats: ...... g	Net Carbs: ...... g Proteins: ...... g Fats: ...... g	....
DINNER	SNACKS	Exercise Type:
		....
		Exercise (Minutes):
Net Carbs: ...... g Proteins: ...... g Fats: ...... g	Net Carbs: ...... g Proteins: ...... g Fats: ...... g	....
DAILY MACROS Net Carbs: ...... g Proteins: ...... g Fats: ...... g		

Notes:

DAY 161 Date: .... Mood Check: 😀 😊 😐 🙁 ☹️

BREAKFAST	LUNCH	Water:
		🥤🥤🥤🥤🥤 🥤🥤🥤🥤🥤
		Sleep (Hours):
Net Carbs: ...... g Proteins: ...... g Fats: ...... g	Net Carbs: ...... g Proteins: ...... g Fats: ...... g	....
DINNER	SNACKS	Exercise Type:
		....
		Exercise (Minutes):
Net Carbs: ...... g Proteins: ...... g Fats: ...... g	Net Carbs: ...... g Proteins: ...... g Fats: ...... g	....
DAILY MACROS Net Carbs: ...... g Proteins: ...... g Fats: ...... g		

Notes:

WEEKLY INTENTIONS

What are you excited for this week?

....

....

....

....

What is something you'd like to work on this week? ....

....

....

....

Carbs: .... %
Proteins: .... %
Fats: .... %

DAY 162   Date: ....   Mood Check: ☺ ☺ ☺ ☹ ☹

BREAKFAST	LUNCH	Water:
		🥛🥛🥛🥛🥛 🥛🥛🥛🥛🥛
		Sleep (Hours):
Net Carbs: ...... g Proteins: ...... g Fats: ...... g	Net Carbs: ...... g Proteins: ...... g Fats: ...... g	....
DINNER	**SNACKS**	Exercise Type:
		....
		Exercise (Minutes):
Net Carbs: ...... g Proteins: ...... g Fats: ...... g	Net Carbs: ...... g Proteins: ...... g Fats: ...... g	....
DAILY MACROS Net Carbs: ...... g Proteins: ...... g Fats: ...... g		

Notes:

DAY 163 Date: .... Mood Check: 🙂 🙂 😐 🙁 ☹️

BREAKFAST	LUNCH	Water:
		🥤🥤🥤🥤🥤 🥤🥤🥤🥤🥤

Net Carbs: ...... g Proteins: ...... g Fats: ...... g | Net Carbs: ...... g Proteins: ...... g Fats: ...... g

Sleep (Hours):
....

DINNER	SNACKS	Exercise Type:
		.... Exercise (Minutes):

Net Carbs: ...... g Proteins: ...... g Fats: ...... g | Net Carbs: ...... g Proteins: ...... g Fats: ...... g

....

DAILY MACROS Net Carbs: ...... g Proteins: ...... g Fats: ...... g

Notes:

DAY 164 Date: .... Mood Check: 🙂 🙂 😐 🙁 ☹️

BREAKFAST	LUNCH	Water:
		🥤🥤🥤🥤🥤 🥤🥤🥤🥤🥤

Net Carbs: ...... g Proteins: ...... g Fats: ...... g | Net Carbs: ...... g Proteins: ...... g Fats: ...... g

Sleep (Hours):
....

DINNER	SNACKS	Exercise Type:
		.... Exercise (Minutes):

Net Carbs: ...... g Proteins: ...... g Fats: ...... g | Net Carbs: ...... g Proteins: ...... g Fats: ...... g

....

DAILY MACROS Net Carbs: ...... g Proteins: ...... g Fats: ...... g

Notes:

DAY 165 Date: .... Mood Check: 😀 😊 😐 🙁 😣

BREAKFAST

LUNCH

Water:

🥛🥛🥛🥛🥛
🥛🥛🥛🥛🥛

Sleep (Hours):

Net Carbs: ...... g Proteins: ...... g Fats: ...... g | Net Carbs: ...... g Proteins: ...... g Fats: ...... g | ....

DINNER

SNACKS

Exercise
Type:

....

Exercise
(Minutes):

Net Carbs: ...... g Proteins: ...... g Fats: ...... g | Net Carbs: ...... g Proteins: ...... g Fats: ...... g

....

DAILY MACROS   Net Carbs: ...... g   Proteins: ...... g   Fats: ...... g

Notes:

DAY 166 Date: .... Mood Check: 😀 😊 😐 🙁 😣

BREAKFAST

LUNCH

Water:

🥛🥛🥛🥛🥛
🥛🥛🥛🥛🥛

Sleep (Hours):

Net Carbs: ...... g Proteins: ...... g Fats: ...... g | Net Carbs: ...... g Proteins: ...... g Fats: ...... g | ....

DINNER

SNACKS

Exercise
Type:

....

Exercise
(Minutes):

Net Carbs: ...... g Proteins: ...... g Fats: ...... g | Net Carbs: ...... g Proteins: ...... g Fats: ...... g

....

DAILY MACROS   Net Carbs: ...... g   Proteins: ...... g   Fats: ...... g

Notes:

DAY 167

Date: .... Mood Check: 😀 🙂 😐 🙁 ☹️

BREAKFAST	LUNCH	Water:
		🥛🥛🥛🥛🥛 🥛🥛🥛🥛🥛
		Sleep (Hours):
Net Carbs: ...... g Proteins: ...... g Fats: ...... g	Net Carbs: ...... g Proteins: ...... g Fats: ...... g	....
DINNER	**SNACKS**	Exercise Type:
		....
		Exercise (Minutes):
Net Carbs: ...... g Proteins: ...... g Fats: ...... g	Net Carbs: ...... g Proteins: ...... g Fats: ...... g	
DAILY MACROS Net Carbs: ...... g Proteins: ...... g Fats: ...... g		....

Notes:

DAY 168

Date: .... Mood Check: 😀 🙂 😐 🙁 ☹️

BREAKFAST	LUNCH	Water:
		🥛🥛🥛🥛🥛 🥛🥛🥛🥛🥛
		Sleep (Hours):
Net Carbs: ...... g Proteins: ...... g Fats: ...... g	Net Carbs: ...... g Proteins: ...... g Fats: ...... g	....
DINNER	**SNACKS**	Exercise Type:
		....
		Exercise (Minutes):
Net Carbs: ...... g Proteins: ...... g Fats: ...... g	Net Carbs: ...... g Proteins: ...... g Fats: ...... g	
DAILY MACROS Net Carbs: ...... g Proteins: ...... g Fats: ...... g		....

Notes:

MEASUREMENT	CURRENT	MONTH CHANGE
WEIGHT (LBS)		
UPPER ARMS (IN)		
CHEST (IN)		
WAIST (IN)		
HIPS (IN)		
THIGHS (IN)		
CALVES (IN)		

CHECKING IN

Congratulations on making it this far! What are you most proud of from the past 4 weeks?

....

....

....

....

....

What was your biggest challenge over the past 4 weeks?

What are some goals you would like to work toward over the next 4 weeks?

Reflect on your mood over the past month—did you notice differences related to your eating habits?

WEEKLY INTENTIONS

What are you excited for this week?

....

....

....

....

Carbs: .... %
Proteins: .... %
Fats: .... %

What is something you'd like to work on this week? ....

....

....

....

DAY 169	Date:	Mood Check: 😀 🙂 😐 🙁 ☹️

BREAKFAST	LUNCH	Water:
		🥛🥛🥛🥛 🥛🥛🥛🥛
		Sleep (Hours):
Net Carbs: ...... g Proteins: ...... g Fats: ...... g	Net Carbs: ...... g Proteins: ...... g Fats: ...... g	....
DINNER	**SNACKS**	Exercise Type: .... Exercise (Minutes):
Net Carbs: ...... g Proteins: ...... g Fats: ...... g	Net Carbs: ...... g Proteins: ...... g Fats: ...... g	....
DAILY MACROS	Net Carbs: ...... g Proteins: ...... g Fats: ...... g	

Notes:

DAY 170   Date: ....   Mood Check: 😊 🙂 😐 🙁 ☹️

BREAKFAST	LUNCH	Water:
		🥤🥤🥤🥤🥤 🥤🥤🥤🥤🥤
Net Carbs: ...... g Proteins: ...... g Fats: ...... g	Net Carbs: ...... g Proteins: ...... g Fats: ...... g	**Sleep (Hours):** ....
DINNER	**SNACKS**	Exercise Type: .... Exercise (Minutes):
Net Carbs: ...... g Proteins: ...... g Fats: ...... g	Net Carbs: ...... g Proteins: ...... g Fats: ...... g	....
DAILY MACROS	Net Carbs: ...... g Proteins: ...... g Fats: ...... g	

Notes:

DAY 171   Date: ....   Mood Check: 😊 🙂 😐 🙁 ☹️

BREAKFAST	LUNCH	Water:
		🥤🥤🥤🥤🥤 🥤🥤🥤🥤🥤
Net Carbs: ...... g Proteins: ...... g Fats: ...... g	Net Carbs: ...... g Proteins: ...... g Fats: ...... g	**Sleep (Hours):** ....
DINNER	**SNACKS**	Exercise Type: .... Exercise (Minutes):
Net Carbs: ...... g Proteins: ...... g Fats: ...... g	Net Carbs: ...... g Proteins: ...... g Fats: ...... g	....
DAILY MACROS	Net Carbs: ...... g Proteins: ...... g Fats: ...... g	

Notes:

DAY 172　Date: ....　Mood Check: 😃 🙂 😐 🙁 😣

BREAKFAST

LUNCH

Water:

Sleep (Hours):

Net Carbs: ...... g Proteins: ...... g Fats: ...... g | Net Carbs: ...... g Proteins: ...... g Fats: ...... g

....

DINNER

SNACKS

Exercise Type:

....

Exercise (Minutes):

Net Carbs: ...... g Proteins: ...... g Fats: ...... g | Net Carbs: ...... g Proteins: ...... g Fats: ...... g

....

DAILY MACROS　Net Carbs: ...... g　Proteins: ...... g　Fats: ...... g

Notes:

DAY 173　Date: ....　Mood Check: 😃 🙂 😐 🙁 😣

BREAKFAST

LUNCH

Water:

Sleep (Hours):

Net Carbs: ...... g Proteins: ...... g Fats: ...... g | Net Carbs: ...... g Proteins: ...... g Fats: ...... g

....

DINNER

SNACKS

Exercise Type:

....

Exercise (Minutes):

Net Carbs: ...... g Proteins: ...... g Fats: ...... g | Net Carbs: ...... g Proteins: ...... g Fats: ...... g

....

DAILY MACROS　Net Carbs: ...... g　Proteins: ...... g　Fats: ...... g

Notes:

DAY 174

Date: .... Mood Check: 😊 🙂 😐 🙁 ☹️

BREAKFAST	LUNCH	Water:
		🥛🥛🥛🥛 🥛🥛🥛🥛
		Sleep (Hours):
Net Carbs: ...... g Proteins: ...... g Fats: ...... g	Net Carbs: ...... g Proteins: ...... g Fats: ...... g	....

DINNER	SNACKS	Exercise Type:
		....
		Exercise (Minutes):
Net Carbs: ...... g Proteins: ...... g Fats: ...... g	Net Carbs: ...... g Proteins: ...... g Fats: ...... g	....

DAILY MACROS   Net Carbs: ...... g   Proteins: ...... g   Fats: ...... g

Notes:

DAY 175

Date: .... Mood Check: 😊 🙂 😐 🙁 ☹️

BREAKFAST	LUNCH	Water:
		🥛🥛🥛🥛 🥛🥛🥛🥛
		Sleep (Hours):
Net Carbs: ...... g Proteins: ...... g Fats: ...... g	Net Carbs: ...... g Proteins: ...... g Fats: ...... g	....

DINNER	SNACKS	Exercise Type:
		....
		Exercise (Minutes):
Net Carbs: ...... g Proteins: ...... g Fats: ...... g	Net Carbs: ...... g Proteins: ...... g Fats: ...... g	....

DAILY MACROS   Net Carbs: ...... g   Proteins: ...... g   Fats: ...... g

Notes:

WEEKLY INTENTIONS

What are you excited for this week?

....

....

....

What is something you'd like to work on this week? ....

....

....

....

Carbs: .... %
Proteins: .... %
Fats: .... %

DAY 176	Date:	Mood Check: ☺ ☺ ☺ ☹ ☹

BREAKFAST

LUNCH

Water:

Net Carbs: ...... g Proteins: ...... g Fats: ...... g

Net Carbs: ...... g Proteins: ...... g Fats: ...... g

Sleep (Hours):

....

DINNER

SNACKS

Exercise Type:

....

Exercise (Minutes):

Net Carbs: ...... g Proteins: ...... g Fats: ...... g

Net Carbs: ...... g Proteins: ...... g Fats: ...... g

....

DAILY MACROS   Net Carbs: ...... g   Proteins: ...... g   Fats: ...... g

Notes:

DAY 177 Date: .... Mood Check: 😀 😊 😐 😟 😣

BREAKFAST	LUNCH	Water:
		🥛🥛🥛🥛 🥛🥛🥛🥛
		Sleep (Hours):
Net Carbs: ...... g Proteins: ...... g Fats: ...... g	Net Carbs: ...... g Proteins: ...... g Fats: ...... g	....
DINNER	**SNACKS**	Exercise Type: .... Exercise (Minutes):
Net Carbs: ...... g Proteins: ...... g Fats: ...... g	Net Carbs: ...... g Proteins: ...... g Fats: ...... g	
DAILY MACROS Net Carbs: ...... g Proteins: ...... g Fats: ...... g		....

Notes:

DAY 178 Date: .... Mood Check: 😀 😊 😐 😟 😣

BREAKFAST	LUNCH	Water:
		🥛🥛🥛🥛🥛 🥛🥛🥛🥛
		Sleep (Hours):
Net Carbs: ...... g Proteins: ...... g Fats: ...... g	Net Carbs: ...... g Proteins: ...... g Fats: ...... g	....
DINNER	**SNACKS**	Exercise Type: .... Exercise (Minutes):
Net Carbs: ...... g Proteins: ...... g Fats: ...... g	Net Carbs: ...... g Proteins: ...... g Fats: ...... g	
DAILY MACROS Net Carbs: ...... g Proteins: ...... g Fats: ...... g		....

Notes:

DAY 179   Date: ....   Mood Check: 😀 🙂 😐 🙁 😞

BREAKFAST	LUNCH	Water:
Net Carbs: ...... g Proteins: ...... g Fats: ...... g	Net Carbs: ...... g Proteins: ...... g Fats: ...... g	Sleep (Hours): ....
DINNER	SNACKS	Exercise Type: ....
Net Carbs: ...... g Proteins: ...... g Fats: ...... g	Net Carbs: ...... g Proteins: ...... g Fats: ...... g	Exercise (Minutes): ....
DAILY MACROS Net Carbs: ...... g Proteins: ...... g Fats: ...... g		

Notes:

DAY 180   Date: ....   Mood Check: 😀 🙂 😐 🙁 😞

BREAKFAST	LUNCH	Water:
Net Carbs: ...... g Proteins: ...... g Fats: ...... g	Net Carbs: ...... g Proteins: ...... g Fats: ...... g	Sleep (Hours): ....
DINNER	SNACKS	Exercise Type: ....
Net Carbs: ...... g Proteins: ...... g Fats: ...... g	Net Carbs: ...... g Proteins: ...... g Fats: ...... g	Exercise (Minutes): ....
DAILY MACROS Net Carbs: ...... g Proteins: ...... g Fats: ...... g		

Notes:

DAY 181

Date: .... Mood Check: 😃 🙂 😐 🙁 😧

BREAKFAST	LUNCH	Water:
		🥛🥛🥛🥛🥛 🥛🥛🥛🥛🥛
		Sleep (Hours):
Net Carbs: ...... g Proteins: ...... g Fats: ...... g	Net Carbs: ...... g Proteins: ...... g Fats: ...... g	....
DINNER	SNACKS	Exercise Type:
		....
		Exercise (Minutes):
Net Carbs: ...... g Proteins: ...... g Fats: ...... g	Net Carbs: ...... g Proteins: ...... g Fats: ...... g	....
DAILY MACROS	Net Carbs: ...... g Proteins: ...... g Fats: ...... g	

Notes:

DAY 182

Date: .... Mood Check: 😃 🙂 😐 🙁 😧

BREAKFAST	LUNCH	Water:
		🥛🥛🥛🥛🥛 🥛🥛🥛🥛🥛
		Sleep (Hours):
Net Carbs: ...... g Proteins: ...... g Fats: ...... g	Net Carbs: ...... g Proteins: ...... g Fats: ...... g	....
DINNER	SNACKS	Exercise Type:
		....
		Exercise (Minutes):
Net Carbs: ...... g Proteins: ...... g Fats: ...... g	Net Carbs: ...... g Proteins: ...... g Fats: ...... g	....
DAILY MACROS	Net Carbs: ...... g Proteins: ...... g Fats: ...... g	

Notes:

WEEKLY INTENTIONS

What are you excited for this week?

....

....

....

....

What is something you'd like to work on this week? ....

....

....

....

DAY 183	Date:	Mood Check: ☺ ☺ 😐 ☹ ☹

BREAKFAST	**LUNCH**	Water:
		🥃🥃🥃🥃🥃 🥃🥃🥃🥃🥃
		Sleep (Hours):
Net Carbs: ...... g Proteins: ...... g Fats: ...... g	Net Carbs: ...... g Proteins: ...... g Fats: ...... g	....
DINNER	**SNACKS**	Exercise Type:
		....
		Exercise (Minutes):
Net Carbs: ...... g Proteins: ...... g Fats: ...... g	Net Carbs: ...... g Proteins: ...... g Fats: ...... g	....
DAILY MACROS	Net Carbs: ...... g Proteins: ...... g Fats: ...... g	

Notes:

DAY 184 Date: .... Mood Check: 😃 😊 😐 🙁 ☹️

BREAKFAST	LUNCH	Water:
		🥛🥛🥛🥛 🥛🥛🥛🥛
		Sleep (Hours):
Net Carbs: ...... g Proteins: ...... g Fats: ...... g	Net Carbs: ...... g Proteins: ...... g Fats: ...... g	....
DINNER	**SNACKS**	Exercise Type:
		....
		Exercise (Minutes):
Net Carbs: ...... g Proteins: ...... g Fats: ...... g	Net Carbs: ...... g Proteins: ...... g Fats: ...... g	
DAILY MACROS Net Carbs: ...... g Proteins: ...... g Fats: ...... g		....

Notes:

DAY 185 Date: .... Mood Check: 😃 😊 😐 🙁 ☹️

BREAKFAST	LUNCH	Water:
		🥛🥛🥛🥛 🥛🥛🥛🥛
		Sleep (Hours):
Net Carbs: ...... g Proteins: ...... g Fats: ...... g	Net Carbs: ...... g Proteins: ...... g Fats: ...... g	....
DINNER	**SNACKS**	Exercise Type:
		....
		Exercise (Minutes):
Net Carbs: ...... g Proteins: ...... g Fats: ...... g	Net Carbs: ...... g Proteins: ...... g Fats: ...... g	
DAILY MACROS Net Carbs: ...... g Proteins: ...... g Fats: ...... g		....

Notes:

DAY 186 Date: .... Mood Check: 😃 😊 😐 🙁 ☹️

BREAKFAST	LUNCH	Water:
		🥤🥤🥤🥤 🥤🥤🥤🥤
		Sleep (Hours):
Net Carbs: ......g Proteins: ......g Fats: ......g	Net Carbs: ......g Proteins: ......g Fats: ......g	....
DINNER	SNACKS	Exercise Type: .... Exercise (Minutes):
Net Carbs: ......g Proteins: ......g Fats: ......g	Net Carbs: ......g Proteins: ......g Fats: ......g	....
DAILY MACROS Net Carbs: ......g Proteins: ......g Fats: ......g		

Notes:

DAY 187 Date: .... Mood Check: 😃 😊 😐 🙁 ☹️

BREAKFAST	LUNCH	Water:
		🥤🥤🥤🥤 🥤🥤🥤🥤
		Sleep (Hours):
Net Carbs: ......g Proteins: ......g Fats: ......g	Net Carbs: ......g Proteins: ......g Fats: ......g	....
DINNER	SNACKS	Exercise Type: .... Exercise (Minutes):
Net Carbs: ......g Proteins: ......g Fats: ......g	Net Carbs: ......g Proteins: ......g Fats: ......g	....
DAILY MACROS Net Carbs: ......g Proteins: ......g Fats: ......g		

Notes:

DAY 188

Date: .... Mood Check: 😃 🙂 😐 🙁 ☹️

BREAKFAST

Net Carbs: ...... g Proteins: ...... g Fats: ...... g

DINNER

Net Carbs: ...... g Proteins: ...... g Fats: ...... g

LUNCH

Net Carbs: ...... g Proteins: ...... g Fats: ...... g

SNACKS

Net Carbs: ...... g Proteins: ...... g Fats: ...... g

Water:

Sleep (Hours):

....

Exercise Type:

....

Exercise (Minutes):

....

DAILY MACROS   Net Carbs: ...... g   Proteins: ...... g   Fats: ...... g

Notes:

DAY 189

Date: .... Mood Check: 😃 🙂 😐 🙁 ☹️

BREAKFAST

Net Carbs: ...... g Proteins: ...... g Fats: ...... g

DINNER

Net Carbs: ...... g Proteins: ...... g Fats: ...... g

LUNCH

Net Carbs: ...... g Proteins: ...... g Fats: ...... g

SNACKS

Net Carbs: ...... g Proteins: ...... g Fats: ...... g

Water:

Sleep (Hours):

....

Exercise Type:

....

Exercise (Minutes):

....

DAILY MACROS   Net Carbs: ...... g   Proteins: ...... g   Fats: ...... g

Notes:

WEEKLY INTENTIONS

What are you excited for this week?

....

....

....

What is something you'd like to work on this week? ....

....

....

....

DAY 190	Date:	Mood Check: 😃 🙂 😐 🙁 ☹️
BREAKFAST	**LUNCH**	Water:
		🥤🥤🥤🥤🥤 🥤🥤🥤🥤🥤
		Sleep (Hours):
Net Carbs: ...... g Proteins: ...... g Fats: ...... g	Net Carbs: ...... g Proteins: ...... g Fats: ...... g	....
DINNER	**SNACKS**	Exercise Type:
		....
		Exercise (Minutes):
Net Carbs: ...... g Proteins: ...... g Fats: ...... g	Net Carbs: ...... g Proteins: ...... g Fats: ...... g	....
DAILY MACROS	Net Carbs: ...... g Proteins: ...... g Fats: ...... g	

Notes:

DAY 191

Date: .... Mood Check: 😀 🙂 😐 🙁 😖

BREAKFAST	LUNCH	Water:
		🥛🥛🥛🥛🥛 🥛🥛🥛🥛🥛
		Sleep (Hours):
Net Carbs: ...... g Proteins: ...... g Fats: ...... g	Net Carbs: ...... g Proteins: ...... g Fats: ...... g	....
DINNER	SNACKS	Exercise Type:
		....
		Exercise (Minutes):
Net Carbs: ...... g Proteins: ...... g Fats: ...... g	Net Carbs: ...... g Proteins: ...... g Fats: ...... g	....
DAILY MACROS	Net Carbs: ...... g Proteins: ...... g Fats: ...... g	

Notes:

DAY 192

Date: .... Mood Check: 😀 🙂 😐 🙁 😖

BREAKFAST	LUNCH	Water:
		🥛🥛🥛🥛🥛 🥛🥛🥛🥛🥛
		Sleep (Hours):
Net Carbs: ...... g Proteins: ...... g Fats: ...... g	Net Carbs: ...... g Proteins: ...... g Fats: ...... g	....
DINNER	SNACKS	Exercise Type:
		....
		Exercise (Minutes):
Net Carbs: ...... g Proteins: ...... g Fats: ...... g	Net Carbs: ...... g Proteins: ...... g Fats: ...... g	....
DAILY MACROS	Net Carbs: ...... g Proteins: ...... g Fats: ...... g	

Notes:

DAY 193 Date: .... Mood Check: 😃 😊 😐 🙁 😫

BREAKFAST	LUNCH	Water:

Net Carbs: ...... g Proteins: ...... g Fats: ...... g | Net Carbs: ...... g Proteins: ...... g Fats: ...... g

Sleep (Hours):
....

DINNER	SNACKS	Exercise Type:

Net Carbs: ...... g Proteins: ...... g Fats: ...... g | Net Carbs: ...... g Proteins: ...... g Fats: ...... g

Exercise (Minutes):
....

DAILY MACROS   Net Carbs: ...... g   Proteins: ...... g   Fats: ...... g

Notes:

DAY 194 Date: .... Mood Check: 😃 😊 😐 🙁 😫

BREAKFAST	LUNCH	Water:

Net Carbs: ...... g Proteins: ...... g Fats: ...... g | Net Carbs: ...... g Proteins: ...... g Fats: ...... g

Sleep (Hours):
....

DINNER	SNACKS	Exercise Type:

Net Carbs: ...... g Proteins: ...... g Fats: ...... g | Net Carbs: ...... g Proteins: ...... g Fats: ...... g

Exercise (Minutes):
....

DAILY MACROS   Net Carbs: ...... g   Proteins: ...... g   Fats: ...... g

Notes:

DAY 195 Date: .... Mood Check: ☺ ☺ 😐 🙁 ☹

BREAKFAST	LUNCH	Water:
		🥤🥤🥤🥤🥤🥤🥤🥤🥤🥤
		Sleep (Hours):
Net Carbs: ...... g Proteins: ...... g Fats: ...... g	Net Carbs: ...... g Proteins: ...... g Fats: ...... g	....
DINNER	**SNACKS**	Exercise Type:
		....
		Exercise (Minutes):
Net Carbs: ...... g Proteins: ...... g Fats: ...... g	Net Carbs: ...... g Proteins: ...... g Fats: ...... g	
DAILY MACROS Net Carbs: ...... g Proteins: ...... g Fats: ...... g		....

Notes:

DAY 196 Date: .... Mood Check: ☺ ☺ 😐 🙁 ☹

BREAKFAST	LUNCH	Water:
		🥤🥤🥤🥤🥤🥤🥤🥤🥤🥤
		Sleep (Hours):
Net Carbs: ...... g Proteins: ...... g Fats: ...... g	Net Carbs: ...... g Proteins: ...... g Fats: ...... g	....
DINNER	**SNACKS**	Exercise Type:
		....
		Exercise (Minutes):
Net Carbs: ...... g Proteins: ...... g Fats: ...... g	Net Carbs: ...... g Proteins: ...... g Fats: ...... g	
DAILY MACROS Net Carbs: ...... g Proteins: ...... g Fats: ...... g		....

Notes:

MEASUREMENT	CURRENT	MONTH CHANGE
WEIGHT (LBS)		
UPPER ARMS (IN)		
CHEST (IN)		
WAIST (IN)		
HIPS (IN)		
THIGHS (IN)		
CALVES (IN)		

CHECKING IN

Congratulations on making it this far! What are you most proud of from the past 4 weeks?

....

....

....

....

....

What was your biggest challenge over the past 4 weeks?

....

....

....

....

....

....

What are some goals you would like to work toward over the next 4 weeks?

....

....

....

....

....

....

Reflect on your mood over the past month—did you notice differences related to your eating habits?

....

....

....

....

....

WEEKLY INTENTIONS

What are you excited for this week?

....

....

....

....

What is something you'd like to work on this week? ....

....

....

....

<table>
<tr><td>TARGET MACROS</td></tr>
<tr><td>Carbs: ....%
Proteins: ....%
Fats: ....%</td></tr>
</table>

DAY 197	Date:	Mood Check: 😀 🙂 😐 🙁 😞

BREAKFAST	LUNCH	Water:
		🥛🥛🥛🥛 🥛🥛🥛🥛
		Sleep (Hours):
Net Carbs: ......g Proteins: ......g Fats: ......g	Net Carbs: ......g Proteins: ......g Fats: ......g	
DINNER	**SNACKS**	Exercise Type: ....
		Exercise (Minutes):
Net Carbs: ......g Proteins: ......g Fats: ......g	Net Carbs: ......g Proteins: ......g Fats: ......g	....
DAILY MACROS	Net Carbs: ......g Proteins: ......g Fats: ......g	

Notes:

DAY 198 Date: .... Mood Check: 😃 😊 😐 🙁 ☹️

BREAKFAST	LUNCH	Water:
		🥤🥤🥤🥤🥤
		🥤🥤🥤🥤🥤
		Sleep (Hours):
Net Carbs: ...... g Proteins: ...... g Fats: ...... g	Net Carbs: ...... g Proteins: ...... g Fats: ...... g	....
DINNER	**SNACKS**	Exercise Type:
		....
		Exercise (Minutes):
Net Carbs: ...... g Proteins: ...... g Fats: ...... g	Net Carbs: ...... g Proteins: ...... g Fats: ...... g	....
DAILY MACROS Net Carbs: .... g Proteins: .... g Fats: .... g		

Notes:

DAY 199 Date: .... Mood Check: 😃 😊 😐 🙁 ☹️

BREAKFAST	LUNCH	Water:
		🥤🥤🥤🥤🥤
		🥤🥤🥤🥤🥤
		Sleep (Hours):
Net Carbs: ...... g Proteins: ...... g Fats: ...... g	Net Carbs: ...... g Proteins: ...... g Fats: ...... g	....
DINNER	**SNACKS**	Exercise Type:
		....
		Exercise (Minutes):
Net Carbs: ...... g Proteins: ...... g Fats: ...... g	Net Carbs: ...... g Proteins: ...... g Fats: ...... g	....
DAILY MACROS Net Carbs: .... g Proteins: .... g Fats: .... g		

Notes:

DAY 200 Date: .... Mood Check: ☺ ☺ ☺ ☹ ☹

BREAKFAST	LUNCH	Water:

Net Carbs: ...... g Proteins: ...... g Fats: ...... g | Net Carbs: ...... g Proteins: ...... g Fats: ...... g

Sleep (Hours):

....

DINNER	SNACKS	Exercise Type:

Exercise (Minutes):

Net Carbs: ...... g Proteins: ...... g Fats: ...... g | Net Carbs: ...... g Proteins: ...... g Fats: ...... g

....

DAILY MACROS   Net Carbs: ...... g   Proteins: ...... g   Fats: ...... g

Notes:

DAY 201 Date: .... Mood Check: ☺ ☺ ☺ ☹ ☹

BREAKFAST	LUNCH	Water:

Net Carbs: ...... g Proteins: ...... g Fats: ...... g | Net Carbs: ...... g Proteins: ...... g Fats: ...... g

Sleep (Hours):

....

DINNER	SNACKS	Exercise Type:

Exercise (Minutes):

Net Carbs: ...... g Proteins: ...... g Fats: ...... g | Net Carbs: ...... g Proteins: ...... g Fats: ...... g

....

DAILY MACROS   Net Carbs: ...... g   Proteins: ...... g   Fats: ...... g

Notes:

DAY 202 Date: .... Mood Check: 😀 😊 😐 🙁 ☹️

BREAKFAST	LUNCH	Water:
		🥛🥛🥛🥛 🥛🥛🥛🥛
		Sleep (Hours):
Net Carbs: ...... g Proteins: ...... g Fats: ...... g	Net Carbs: ...... g Proteins: ...... g Fats: ...... g	....

DINNER	SNACKS	Exercise Type:
		....
		Exercise (Minutes):
Net Carbs: ...... g Proteins: ...... g Fats: ...... g	Net Carbs: ...... g Proteins: ...... g Fats: ...... g	....

DAILY MACROS   Net Carbs: ...... g   Proteins: ...... g   Fats: ...... g

Notes:

DAY 203 Date: .... Mood Check: 😀 😊 😐 🙁 ☹️

BREAKFAST	LUNCH	Water:
		🥛🥛🥛🥛 🥛🥛🥛🥛
		Sleep (Hours):
Net Carbs: ...... g Proteins: ...... g Fats: ...... g	Net Carbs: ...... g Proteins: ...... g Fats: ...... g	....

DINNER	SNACKS	Exercise Type:
		....
		Exercise (Minutes):
Net Carbs: ...... g Proteins: ...... g Fats: ...... g	Net Carbs: ...... g Proteins: ...... g Fats: ...... g	....

DAILY MACROS   Net Carbs: ...... g   Proteins: ...... g   Fats: ...... g

Notes:

WEEKLY INTENTIONS

What are you excited for this week?

Carbs: .... %
Proteins: .... %
Fats: .... %

....

....

....

....

What is something you'd like to work on this week? ....

....

....

....

DAY 204   Date: ....   Mood Check: 😀 😊 😐 🙁 😞

BREAKFAST	LUNCH	Water:
		🥤🥤🥤🥤🥤 🥤🥤🥤🥤🥤
		Sleep (Hours):
Net Carbs: ...... g Proteins: ...... g Fats: ...... g	Net Carbs: ...... g Proteins: ...... g Fats: ...... g	....
DINNER	**SNACKS**	Exercise Type:
		....
		Exercise (Minutes):
Net Carbs: ...... g Proteins: ...... g Fats: ...... g	Net Carbs: ...... g Proteins: ...... g Fats: ...... g	....

DAILY MACROS   Net Carbs: ...... g   Proteins: ...... g   Fats: ...... g

Notes:

DAY 205 Date: .... Mood Check: 😃 ☺ 😐 🙁 ☹

BREAKFAST	LUNCH	Water:
		🥛🥛🥛🥛 🥛🥛🥛🥛
		Sleep (Hours):
Net Carbs: ...... g Proteins: ...... g Fats: ...... g	Net Carbs: ...... g Proteins: ...... g Fats: ...... g	....
DINNER	**SNACKS**	Exercise Type:
		....
		Exercise (Minutes):
Net Carbs: ...... g Proteins: ...... g Fats: ...... g	Net Carbs: ...... g Proteins: ...... g Fats: ...... g	....
DAILY MACROS Net Carbs: ...... g Proteins: ...... g Fats: ...... g		

Notes:

DAY 206 Date: .... Mood Check: 😃 ☺ 😐 🙁 ☹

BREAKFAST	LUNCH	Water:
		🥛🥛🥛🥛 🥛🥛🥛🥛
		Sleep (Hours):
Net Carbs: ...... g Proteins: ...... g Fats: ...... g	Net Carbs: ...... g Proteins: ...... g Fats: ...... g	....
DINNER	**SNACKS**	Exercise Type:
		....
		Exercise (Minutes):
Net Carbs: ...... g Proteins: ...... g Fats: ...... g	Net Carbs: ...... g Proteins: ...... g Fats: ...... g	....
DAILY MACROS Net Carbs: ...... g Proteins: ...... g Fats: ...... g		

Notes:

DAY 207

Date: .... Mood Check: 😃 🙂 😐 🙁 ☹️

BREAKFAST

LUNCH

Net Carbs: ...... g Proteins: ...... g Fats: ...... g | Net Carbs: ...... g Proteins: ...... g Fats: ...... g

DINNER

SNACKS

Net Carbs: ...... g Proteins: ...... g Fats: ...... g | Net Carbs: ...... g Proteins: ...... g Fats: ...... g

DAILY MACROS   Net Carbs: ...... g   Proteins: ...... g   Fats: ...... g

Water:

Sleep (Hours):

Exercise Type:

Exercise (Minutes):

Notes:

DAY 208

Date: .... Mood Check: 😃 🙂 😐 🙁 ☹️

BREAKFAST

LUNCH

Net Carbs: ...... g Proteins: ...... g Fats: ...... g | Net Carbs: ...... g Proteins: ...... g Fats: ...... g

DINNER

SNACKS

Net Carbs: ...... g Proteins: ...... g Fats: ...... g | Net Carbs: ...... g Proteins: ...... g Fats: ...... g

DAILY MACROS   Net Carbs: ...... g   Proteins: ...... g   Fats: ...... g

Water:

Sleep (Hours):

Exercise Type:

Exercise (Minutes):

Notes:

DAY 209 — Date: .... Mood Check: 😃 😊 😐 🙁 😣

BREAKFAST	LUNCH	Water:
		🥤🥤🥤🥤 🥤🥤🥤🥤
		Sleep (Hours):
Net Carbs: ...... g Proteins: ...... g Fats: ...... g	Net Carbs: ...... g Proteins: ...... g Fats: ...... g	....

DINNER	SNACKS	Exercise Type:
		....
		Exercise (Minutes):
Net Carbs: ...... g Proteins: ...... g Fats: ...... g	Net Carbs: ...... g Proteins: ...... g Fats: ...... g	....

DAILY MACROS   Net Carbs: ...... g   Proteins: ...... g   Fats: ...... g

Notes:

DAY 210 — Date: .... Mood Check: 😃 😊 😐 🙁 😣

BREAKFAST	LUNCH	Water:
		🥤🥤🥤🥤 🥤🥤🥤🥤
		Sleep (Hours):
Net Carbs: ...... g Proteins: ...... g Fats: ...... g	Net Carbs: ...... g Proteins: ...... g Fats: ...... g	....

DINNER	SNACKS	Exercise Type:
		....
		Exercise (Minutes):
Net Carbs: ...... g Proteins: ...... g Fats: ...... g	Net Carbs: ...... g Proteins: ...... g Fats: ...... g	....

DAILY MACROS   Net Carbs: ...... g   Proteins: ...... g   Fats: ...... g

Notes:

WEEKLY INTENTIONS

What are you excited for this week?

....

....

....

....

What is something you'd like to work on this week? ....

....

....

....

TARGET MACROS

Carbs:	...........%
Proteins:	...........%
Fats:	...........%

DAY 211

Date: .... Mood Check: 😀 🙂 😐 🙁 😣

BREAKFAST	LUNCH	Water:
		🥤🥤🥤🥤🥤 🥤🥤🥤🥤🥤
		Sleep (Hours):
Net Carbs: ......g Proteins: ......g Fats: ......g	Net Carbs: ......g Proteins: ......g Fats: ......g	....
DINNER	SNACKS	Exercise Type:
		....
		Exercise (Minutes):
Net Carbs: ......g Proteins: ......g Fats: ......g	Net Carbs: ......g Proteins: ......g Fats: ......g	....
DAILY MACROS	Net Carbs: ......g Proteins: ......g Fats: ......g	

Notes:

DAY 2I2

Date: .... Mood Check: 😀 😊 😐 😕 😣

BREAKFAST	LUNCH	Water:
		🥤🥤🥤🥤 🥤🥤🥤🥤
		Sleep (Hours):
Net Carbs: ...... g Proteins: ...... g Fats: ...... g	Net Carbs: ...... g Proteins: ...... g Fats: ...... g	....
DINNER	**SNACKS**	Exercise Type:
		....
		Exercise (Minutes):
Net Carbs: ...... g Proteins: ...... g Fats: ...... g	Net Carbs: ...... g Proteins: ...... g Fats: ...... g	....
DAILY MACROS Net Carbs: .... g Proteins: .... g Fats: .... g		

Notes:

DAY 2I3

Date: .... Mood Check: 😀 😊 😐 😕 😣

BREAKFAST	LUNCH	Water:
		🥤🥤🥤🥤 🥤🥤🥤🥤
		Sleep (Hours):
Net Carbs: ...... g Proteins: ...... g Fats: ...... g	Net Carbs: ...... g Proteins: ...... g Fats: ...... g	....
DINNER	**SNACKS**	Exercise Type:
		....
		Exercise (Minutes):
Net Carbs: ...... g Proteins: ...... g Fats: ...... g	Net Carbs: ...... g Proteins: ...... g Fats: ...... g	....
DAILY MACROS Net Carbs: .... g Proteins: .... g Fats: .... g		

Notes:

DAY 214

Date: .... Mood Check: 😄 😊 😐 🙁 😣

BREAKFAST	LUNCH	Water:
		🥛🥛🥛🥛🥛 🥛🥛🥛🥛🥛
		Sleep (Hours):
Net Carbs: ...... g Proteins: ...... g Fats: ...... g	Net Carbs: ...... g Proteins: ...... g Fats: ...... g	....
DINNER	SNACKS	Exercise Type:
		....
		Exercise (Minutes):
Net Carbs: ...... g Proteins: ...... g Fats: ...... g	Net Carbs: ...... g Proteins: ...... g Fats: ...... g	....
DAILY MACROS Net Carbs: ...... g Proteins: ...... g Fats: ...... g		

Notes:

DAY 215

Date: .... Mood Check: 😄 😊 😐 🙁 😣

BREAKFAST	LUNCH	Water:
		🥛🥛🥛🥛🥛 🥛🥛🥛🥛🥛
		Sleep (Hours):
Net Carbs: ...... g Proteins: ...... g Fats: ...... g	Net Carbs: ...... g Proteins: ...... g Fats: ...... g	....
DINNER	SNACKS	Exercise Type:
		....
		Exercise (Minutes):
Net Carbs: ...... g Proteins: ...... g Fats: ...... g	Net Carbs: ...... g Proteins: ...... g Fats: ...... g	....
DAILY MACROS Net Carbs: ...... g Proteins: ...... g Fats: ...... g		

Notes:

DAY 216   Date: ....   Mood Check: 😃 😊 😐 🙁 😣

BREAKFAST	LUNCH	Water:
		🥛🥛🥛🥛🥛 🥛🥛🥛🥛🥛
		Sleep (Hours):
Net Carbs: ...... g Proteins: ...... g Fats: ...... g	Net Carbs: ...... g Proteins: ...... g Fats: ...... g	....
DINNER	**SNACKS**	Exercise Type: .... Exercise (Minutes):
Net Carbs: ...... g Proteins: ...... g Fats: ...... g	Net Carbs: ...... g Proteins: ...... g Fats: ...... g	....

DAILY MACROS   Net Carbs: .... g   Proteins: .... g   Fats: .... g

Notes:

DAY 217   Date: ....   Mood Check: 😃 😊 😐 🙁 😣

BREAKFAST	LUNCH	Water:
		🥛🥛🥛🥛🥛 🥛🥛🥛🥛🥛
		Sleep (Hours):
Net Carbs: ...... g Proteins: ...... g Fats: ...... g	Net Carbs: ...... g Proteins: ...... g Fats: ...... g	....
DINNER	**SNACKS**	Exercise Type: .... Exercise (Minutes):
Net Carbs: ...... g Proteins: ...... g Fats: ...... g	Net Carbs: ...... g Proteins: ...... g Fats: ...... g	....

DAILY MACROS   Net Carbs: .... g   Proteins: .... g   Fats: .... g

Notes:

WEEKLY INTENTIONS

What are you excited for this week?

....

....

....

....

What is something you'd like to work on this week? ....

....

....

....

DAY 218	Date:	Mood Check: 😀 😊 😐 🙁 ☹️

BREAKFAST	LUNCH	Water:
		🥤🥤🥤🥤🥤 🥤🥤🥤🥤🥤
		Sleep (Hours):
Net Carbs: ......g Proteins: ......g Fats: ......g	Net Carbs: ......g Proteins: ......g Fats: ......g	....
DINNER	SNACKS	Exercise Type:
		Exercise (Minutes):
Net Carbs: ......g Proteins: ......g Fats: ......g	Net Carbs: ......g Proteins: ......g Fats: ......g	....
DAILY MACROS	Net Carbs: ......g Proteins: ......g Fats: ......g	

Notes: ....

DAY 219 Date: .... Mood Check: 😊 😊 😐 😕 😣

BREAKFAST	LUNCH	Water:
		🥛🥛🥛🥛🥛 🥛🥛🥛🥛🥛
		Sleep (Hours):
Net Carbs: ...... g Proteins: ...... g Fats: ...... g	Net Carbs: ...... g Proteins: ...... g Fats: ...... g	....
DINNER	SNACKS	Exercise Type:
		....
		Exercise (Minutes):
Net Carbs: ...... g Proteins: ...... g Fats: ...... g	Net Carbs: ...... g Proteins: ...... g Fats: ...... g	....

DAILY MACROS   Net Carbs: ...... g   Proteins: ...... g   Fats: ...... g

Notes:

DAY 220 Date: .... Mood Check: 😊 😊 😐 😕 😣

BREAKFAST	LUNCH	Water:
		🥛🥛🥛🥛🥛 🥛🥛🥛🥛🥛
		Sleep (Hours):
Net Carbs: ...... g Proteins: ...... g Fats: ...... g	Net Carbs: ...... g Proteins: ...... g Fats: ...... g	....
DINNER	SNACKS	Exercise Type:
		....
		Exercise (Minutes):
Net Carbs: ...... g Proteins: ...... g Fats: ...... g	Net Carbs: ...... g Proteins: ...... g Fats: ...... g	....

DAILY MACROS   Net Carbs: ...... g   Proteins: ...... g   Fats: ...... g

Notes:

DAY 221 Date: .... Mood Check: 😃 😊 😐 😟 😠

BREAKFAST	LUNCH	Water:
		🥤🥤🥤🥤🥤 🥤🥤🥤🥤🥤
		Sleep (Hours):
Net Carbs: ...... g Proteins: ...... g Fats: ...... g	Net Carbs: ...... g Proteins: ...... g Fats: ...... g	....
DINNER	**SNACKS**	Exercise Type:
		....
		Exercise (Minutes):
Net Carbs: ...... g Proteins: ...... g Fats: ...... g	Net Carbs: ...... g Proteins: ...... g Fats: ...... g	
DAILY MACROS Net Carbs: .... g Proteins: .... g Fats: .... g		....

Notes:

DAY 222 Date: .... Mood Check: 😃 😊 😐 😟 😠

BREAKFAST	LUNCH	Water:
		🥤🥤🥤🥤🥤 🥤🥤🥤🥤🥤
		Sleep (Hours):
Net Carbs: ...... g Proteins: ...... g Fats: ...... g	Net Carbs: ...... g Proteins: ...... g Fats: ...... g	....
DINNER	**SNACKS**	Exercise Type:
		....
		Exercise (Minutes):
Net Carbs: ...... g Proteins: ...... g Fats: ...... g	Net Carbs: ...... g Proteins: ...... g Fats: ...... g	
DAILY MACROS Net Carbs: .... g Proteins: .... g Fats: .... g		....

Notes:

DAY 223 Date: .... Mood Check: 😀 😊 😐 🙁 😞

BREAKFAST	LUNCH	Water:
		🥛🥛🥛🥛 🥛🥛🥛🥛
		Sleep (Hours):
Net Carbs: ...... g Proteins: ...... g Fats: ...... g	Net Carbs: ...... g Proteins: ...... g Fats: ...... g	....
DINNER	SNACKS	Exercise Type: .... Exercise (Minutes):
Net Carbs: ...... g Proteins: ...... g Fats: ...... g	Net Carbs: ...... g Proteins: ...... g Fats: ...... g	....
DAILY MACROS	Net Carbs: ...... g Proteins: ...... g Fats: ...... g	

Notes:

DAY 224 Date: .... Mood Check: 😀 😊 😐 🙁 😞

BREAKFAST	LUNCH	Water:
		🥛🥛🥛🥛 🥛🥛🥛🥛
		Sleep (Hours):
Net Carbs: ...... g Proteins: ...... g Fats: ...... g	Net Carbs: ...... g Proteins: ...... g Fats: ...... g	....
DINNER	SNACKS	Exercise Type: .... Exercise (Minutes):
Net Carbs: ...... g Proteins: ...... g Fats: ...... g	Net Carbs: ...... g Proteins: ...... g Fats: ...... g	....
DAILY MACROS	Net Carbs: ...... g Proteins: ...... g Fats: ...... g	

Notes:

MEASUREMENT	CURRENT	MONTH CHANGE
WEIGHT (LBS)		
UPPER ARMS (IN)		
CHEST (IN)		
WAIST (IN)		
HIPS (IN)		
THIGHS (IN)		
CALVES (IN)		

CHECKING IN

Congratulations on making it this far! What are you most proud of from the past 4 weeks?

....

....

....

....

....

What was your biggest challenge over the past 4 weeks?

....

....

....

....

....

What are some goals you would like to work toward over the next 4 weeks?

....

....

....

....

....

Reflect on your mood over the past month—did you notice differences related to your eating habits?

....

....

....

....

....